6-Minute Fitness at 60+

2021

Step by step Guide to doing simple home exercises to recover strength, balance and Energy in 15 days

Table of Contents

Introduction

If you're 60 or older, the thought of becoming frail, suffering injuries from falls, and losing your independence is often a real worry, even if it isn't already happening. Our body changes as we age—and often in ways we don't like. We naturally lose 1–2 percent of our lean muscle mass every year after the age of 50. This gradual loss of muscle and strength is barely noticeable at first—until we wake up one day surprised that our physical ability is not what it used to be.

What if I could show you how to reverse muscle loss and reclaim your strength, balance, and energy faster than you ever thought possible?

What if I gave you a science-based, field-tested approach to exercise that takes only six minutes, twice a day … and what if you could see dramatic results in just the first 15 days?

It doesn't matter if you're 60 or 100 years old, or if you've been active or inactive your entire life. It doesn't matter if you're currently walking miles every day or struggling just to get up from a chair. It doesn't even matter if your health is perfect or imperfect. This book will show you how to transform your body and your life, no matter who you are, irrespective of your current state of health and fitness.

How I Can Help

I'm Dr. Jonathan Su, physical therapist.

Throughout my career, I've worked one-on-one with over 10,000 clients from ages 3 to 103, have read thousands of pages of scientific literature, and tried just about every type of treatment, technique, and exercise program you can imagine. I've even co-authored some of the research myself and wrote a textbook (translated into five languages) that teaches healthcare professionals how to evaluate and treat physical dysfunction wherever it shows up in the body.

At this point, I can confidently say that while I don't know everything, I know what works and what doesn't.

Building a stronger and more capable body isn't nearly as difficult or complicated as everyone imagines. You don't need to toil away hours every week for months on end to see changes. You don't need a ton of different exercises, fancy gym equipment, or complicated movements to achieve great results.

The real science to reversing age-related muscle loss and to rebuilding your body is simple, much simpler than most people realize. No matter who you are, you have the power to transform your body and your life.

What You Will Learn

- A straightforward, science-based exercise plan that only takes six minutes, twice a day and produces consistent strengthening and mobility improvements.

- Three simple bodyweight exercises that effectively target the muscle groups you need to stay active, prevent falls, and remain independent.

- How to design workouts at home that don't rely on complicated equipment.

- The seven most important strategies for benefiting from regular workouts.

- How to develop a winning mindset to help you stay motivated and be consistent with exercise.

- Practical advice and guidance for family members and caregivers helping aging adults with exercise.

Imagine waking up every morning and feeling excited because you know your body is finally working with you, not against you. Imagine feeling more capable and confident in your body and ready to get other parts of your life under control. Imagine doing all the things you want to do and not having to worry about being hampered down by a lack of energy.

You can have all these things, and it's easier than you think.

Just ask Deborah, who had just turned 90 when I met her and had become frail during a recent hospitalization. She had to sleep on the couch in her living room because she was too weak to climb up the stairs to her second-floor bedroom. Less than a week after beginning this program, she literally threw away her walker because she didn't need it anymore. After two weeks, she was sleeping in her bed again because the stairs were no longer an issue.

You can also ask Frank, a healthy, active 68-year-old retired software engineer who noticed that his golf game was suffering due to age-related changes in his body. He was surprised to learn that walking two miles every morning with his wife wasn't enough to keep up his strength. A few weeks after starting this program, his golf game had improved to a level he hadn't reached in over a decade. He was also having a ton more fun with his three grandchildren because he was feeling stronger and more energetic than ever before.

Deborah and Frank are people just like you. If they could change their body and their life, you can too.

My Promise to You

I've worked with thousands of other older adults using the same program you're about to learn in this book. They have consistently amazed themselves, their families, and their doctors with their results, and their lives have been changed by my work. After applying the knowledge in this book, they move and feel better than ever before. They are the proof that this book can help you move and feel your best.

Here's my promise to you. If you follow the program in this book exactly as I lay it out, I guarantee you will experience dramatic improvements in your strength, balance, and energy in as little as 15 days.

Don't be the person who waits until it's too late to take action; be the one who acts immediately to take care of problems before they become bigger issues. Don't be the person who misses out on life's opportunities because of physical limitations; be the one who makes the necessary changes to live a full life. Don't be the person whose loved ones constantly worry about them; be one other people marvel at and say, "I don't know how they do it."

If you've read this far, you've already taken a leap toward a new you — a you that is stronger and more capable, a you with more vigor and energy than anyone thought possible.

Turn to the next page right now and begin your journey to the life-changing transformation that awaits.

Part 1:
Five Things We Never Learned About Exercise for Older Adults

Knowledge is power. You can rest assured knowing that everything I'm about to share with you here is backed by scientific research.

My goal is to empower you with accurate, up-to-date information, which I hope will get you excited about the journey you're embarking on toward a fitter, happier, and healthier you.

Part 1 Topics:

- You can build lean muscle and strength at any age.

- Fitness is a fountain of youth that slows aging and optimizes health.

- Exercise for six minutes, twice daily, to create dramatic changes in 15 days.

- Achieve great results at home with little or no workout equipment.

- Walking does not reverse age-related muscle loss.

1. You Can Build Muscle and Strength at Any Age

I want to debunk the common belief that we are destined to get weak and frail as we age.

Take the case of Charles Eugster, a retired dentist who was sedentary for most of his adult life. In his 80s, he found that his body had deteriorated: his muscles had slackened, he had lost most of his strength, and he had a "pancake butt," as he puts it. "I looked in the mirror one morning, and I didn't like what I saw."

That spurred Charles to take up strength training for the first time in his life, at 87 years old. To his surprise, he soon noticed changes and completely rebuilt his body within a few years. Feeling healthier and stronger than ever, he decided to take up running in his 90s, and in 2015, aged 95, he broke the 200-meter world record for his age group at the British Masters Indoor Track & Field Championships.

Eugster wrote, "People have been brainwashed to think that after you're 65, you're finished. We're told that old age is a continuous state of decline and that we should stop working, slow down and prepare to die. I disagree."[1]

Of course, the human body does change as we age, and often in ways we don't like. As we get older, we begin to lose lean muscle mass and strength. Age-related muscle loss is medically referred to as sarcopenia, a term derived from the Latin words "sarco" for muscle and "penia" for wasting. We naturally lose 3–5 percent of our muscle mass every decade after the age of 30 if we don't take steps to prevent it. This process accelerates after age 50 when we start to lose about 1–2 percent of our muscles every year! Over time, this loss of muscle and strength can lead to frailty, disability, and decreased function. It also increases the risk of falls, one of the most common reasons older adults end up in the hospital.

In the past, scientists believed that it was impossible to improve bodily functions in the elderly and we were destined to decline in function as we grew older. Some of these beliefs are still commonly held today. But recent studies find these assumptions to be untrue; in fact, they couldn't be further from the truth. No matter your age, you can increase strength and lean muscle mass through strength training.

Research published in Medicine & Science in Sports & Exercise analyzed data from 49 studies, representing 1,328 adults over the age of 50 whose muscle mass was shown to increase by an average of nearly a half pound per month with strength exercises.[2] Not only did the exercise reverse muscle loss in older adults, it actually built a lot of new muscle!

Related research found that the intensity of strengthening programs dramatically influenced outcomes. Older adults who participated in higher-intensity programs have been shown to boost their strength by nearly a third more compared to lower-intensity programs.[3]

According to Dr. Marcas Bamman, PhD, director of the University of Alabama at Birmingham Center for Exercise Medicine, scientific studies have repeatedly shown that older muscles can grow and strengthen. In his studies, men and women in their 60s and 70s who began strength training developed muscles that were as large and strong as those of the average 40-year-old.[4]

Clearly, the time in which we say that older adults can't improve is long gone. The story of Charles Eugster and dozens of new research studies make it clear that you can rebuild your body at any age. But the benefits of exercise go far beyond improving strength and physical function. Research shows that exercise can actually slow the aging process and optimize health.

Action Steps

- Take your age and subtract 50. Now multiply the number you get by 2. The result is the percentage of muscle mass you may have lost since you were 50 years old if you haven't consistently been on a strength training program.

2. Fitness: A Fountain of Youth that Slows Aging and Optimizes Health

We've always known that exercise is good for our body and can help us maintain a healthy weight. But we don't always know the specifics of exactly what it does for us. Besides making our body stronger and helping us maintain a healthy weight, exercise can slow the aging process and optimize our health.

Slow the Aging Process

In numerous studies, physical activity has been associated with alterations in telomere length, an indicator of biological aging.[5] Telomeres are the caps at the end of each strand of DNA that protect our chromosomes. Just as the plastic tips on the ends of shoelaces keep the laces from fraying, telomeres prevent chromosomes from fraying or tangling with one another. Think of them as a biological clock that affects how our cells age. Every time a cell divides, the telomeres get shorter, causing us to age and be more vulnerable to diseases such as heart disease, diabetes, and cancer. When the telomeres get too short, the cell can no longer divide and dies.

The good part? Longer telomeres slow down the aging process and are associated with health and longevity—and studies show that the more physically active you are, the longer your telomeres. People who exercised the most had telomeres similar in length to inactive people who were up to 10 years younger.[6] Research also suggests that exercise may be more important than genes when it comes to keeping people young. A study looking at a group of 2,401 twins showed that when one twin was sedentary and the other was active, the active twin had longer telomeres.[7] Investigators have found that higher-intensity activity is associated with longer telomere length, even in older adults.[8] Thus, people who exercise regularly tend to look and feel younger than their actual age, and now research may be able to explain it at a cellular level.

Optimize Health

So many scientific studies have accumulated over the last two decades that the incredible benefits of exercise are now indisputable.[9]

Here's a summary of the science-backed ways exercise can lead to a happier, healthier you:

- **Improve mood and lower depression:** When you exercise, your body releases endorphins that can improve your mood, reduce stress, ward off anxiety and depression, and make you feel more relaxed.

- **Reduce chronic pain:** Exercise has been shown to decrease inflammation and overall pain levels with no additional medication.

- **Keep your brain sharp and lower the risk of dementia:** Exercise stimulates your body to release proteins and other chemicals that improve thinking, learning, and judgment skills as you age. And research shows it keeps dementia at bay and eases some of its symptoms for those who already have it.

- **Improve sexual function:** In men, exercise can improve sexual function and reduce the effects of erectile dysfunction. In women, exercise may increase sexual arousal.

- **Reduce blood pressure and the risk of heart disease:** Regular exercise strengthens your heart and improves circulation, which helps reduce the risk of high cholesterol, coronary artery disease, and heart attack. Exercise can also lower your blood pressure and triglyceride levels.

- **Strengthen your bones:** We already know that exercise can build muscle and strength in older adults. Exercise can also prevent the loss of bone density (osteoporosis) that comes with aging.

- **Reduce your risk of cancer:** Exercise has been shown to reduce the risk of breast, uterine, <u>colon</u>, and <u>lung</u> cancers.

- **Improve your sleep:** Exercise can help you fall asleep faster and stay asleep longer.

- **Reduce your risk of falls:** Research shows that exercise can improve balance and help reduce your risk of falling.

- **Control weight:** Along with diet, exercise plays an important role in preventing obesity and helping you to lose weight.

- **Speedy recovery from illness or injury:** Regular exercise by older adults may decrease the time it takes for a wound to heal by 25 percent. Also, a fit body can better fight off infection and recover more easily from illness or injury.

- **Manage blood sugar and insulin level:** Exercise can reduce your risk for metabolic syndrome and type 2 diabetes by lowering your <u>blood sugar</u> and helping your insulin work better. If you already have one of those diseases, exercise can help you better manage it.

As you can see, the benefits of exercise go far beyond improving strength and physical function. In addition to building a stronger and more capable body, exercise will also change your overall health, longevity, and quality of life in powerful ways.

Action Steps

- Look at the list of science-backed ways exercise can lead to a happier, healthier you, and make a list of the ones that apply to you. Then, think about how your life would be better if exercise improved just a few of the issues on your list.

3. Six Minutes, Twice Daily; Dramatic Changes in 15 Days

Everyone has heard the old adage, "Work smarter, not harder." In fitness terms, this can be more appropriately revised to "Work smarter, not longer," and nowhere is this concept more applicable than with fitness for older adults. By working smart, you can reap the benefits of exercise in as little as six minutes. Yes—six.

I'd like to share with you a true story about a 75-year-old client of mine, Evelyn, from San Francisco, CA.

Soon after returning from a trip to New York City in March 2020, Evelyn began to experience fever, fatigue, and body aches. "At first I thought I had the flu, but then I started having difficulty breathing." Evelyn was rushed to the emergency room and subsequently spent 45 days on a ventilator with a diagnosis of COVID-19. "It was the worst experience of my life being on the verge of death, feeling so helpless, and knowing that my family was worried sick about me."

Thankfully, Evelyn pulled through and was released. The day after her release, her family asked me to visit her at home. This once active and energetic person who loved gardening couldn't walk 10 feet without struggling. Obviously, COVID-19 and its aftermath had taken a toll on her. She reported, "Standing up from a chair felt like I had a 500-pound gorilla on my back. Walking 20 steps from my bedroom to the kitchen felt like a marathon, even with a walker and my daughter helping me."

I immediately started her on the six-minute, twice daily program, and she was soon walking without assistance. "I couldn't believe it! I got rid of the walker in two weeks, started gardening again in four weeks, and felt stronger than I was 15 years ago in eight weeks."

Evelyn is only one of the thousands of older adults who have changed their life with this program. How did we rebuild Evelyn's function so quickly—and how can you do the same?

High-Intensity Interval Training

Six minutes doesn't sound like enough time to make a difference, but the results of over a dozen high-quality studies have found that short bouts of higher-intensity exercise are a more potent method of improving fitness in older adults than traditional forms of exercise.[10]

Many of these studies have focused on a form of exercise known as High-Intensity Interval Training (HIIT). The words "high intensity" may sound scary, but you have nothing to fear. HIIT is a simple concept.

You work harder than you're used to for 30 seconds or even a couple of minutes. And then, after you catch your breath, you can do it again. During a HIIT workout, you alternate between exerting high-level and low-level effort.

Japanese researcher Dr. Izumi Tabata was among the first to recognize the special benefits of high-intensity training. While studying the workout routines of Olympic speed skaters in the mid-1990s, he was surprised to discover that those who performed four minutes of higher-intensity exercise produced better results than those who performed an hour of lower-intensity exercise.

HIIT has been intensively studied since Dr. Tabata made his discovery, and researchers have found that it can improve health and fitness for just about everyone. What's more, higher-intensity exercise is safe and more effective than traditional exercise for people with cardiovascular disease, respiratory disease, heart failure, obesity, diabetes, stroke, and cancer.[11] Higher-intensity exercise has also demonstrated its safety for people over 60 who are untrained and sedentary.[12] Additionally, HIIT improves aerobic endurance and muscle capacity rapidly and dramatically; remarkably, participants in one study more than doubled their "time until exhaustion" on an endurance test after only two weeks of HIIT.[13]

While the benefits are great, you should watch out for a few potential downsides. Because it requires you to push harder than you're used to, be sure to listen to your body and ease up on exercise if needed. HIIT can affect balance for up to 30 minutes following a workout, so caution is advised after exercise to reduce the risk of falls. Finally, sedentary individuals with underlying cardiovascular disease are at a higher risk for complications with higher-intensity physical activities, so it's a good idea to get clearance from your doctor beforehand.

Overall, though, the research shows that higher-intensity exercise is safe for older adults and more effective than traditional exercise despite a substantially lower time commitment and volume of exercise. This is true even for sedentary, untrained older adults who are dealing with a variety of health conditions.

One thing I'd like to clarify is that high-intensity is not the same as high-impact. High-impact exercises—such as prolonged walking on hard surfaces, hiking down inclines, and running—put a lot of stress on your joints. Those activities are not high-intensity exercises like the ones you'll learn in this book. "High-intensity" simply means that you're exerting a higher level of effort, pushing yourself harder than you're used to; the exercise doesn't have to be high-impact.

By adapting the scientific research on higher-intensity exercise to make these activities safe and effective for older adults, I have enabled you to reclaim your body's function and improve your life in just a couple of weeks. And although HIIT requires you to alternate between high- and low-intensity levels of exercise, you actually don't have to worry about this alternation during the exercises described in this book because I've designed the program to make that happen automatically.

The best part is that you don't even need to go to a gym because you can get the same benefits with this program at home, using little or no equipment. We'll explore this more in depth in the next chapter.

Action Steps

- Make an appointment with your primary care provider so you can get cleared to begin this program. Take this book with you to show them the exercise illustrations in part 4 and the exercise schedule in part 5. Your primary care provider may clear you for all the exercises or may limit you to certain ones.

4. Great Results at Home with Little or No Equipment

During the coronavirus pandemic, workout equipment flew off the shelves, with millions of people scrambling to put together a home gym because fitness centers were closing across the country. Equipment such as weights, exercise bikes, and rowers were out of stock for months. The good news is exercise can be just as effective without a gym or workout equipment. You can easily achieve the same results—or even better—exercising at home with little or no workout equipment using something called "functional training."

Functional Training

Functional training mimics activities or specific skills you perform at home, at work, or in sports to help you thrive in your daily life. This kind of training is effective because it uses different muscles simultaneously and also emphasizes core stability — the control of muscles around the abdomen and back that protect your spine when you move. For example, performing squats with a chair trains the same muscles you use when you rise from a chair, pick up an object from the ground, climb stairs, or hike up a mountain.

Many fitness and rehabilitation experts, including myself, have known for a while that functional training is the most effective way to train. Finally, the research is catching up with our observations. Functional training has now been shown in multiple studies to produce results that are superior to most other forms of exercise for diverse groups of people, including young military personnel, middle-aged females with low back pain, and (of course) older adults.[14]

One study demonstrated that high-intensity functional training was safe and effective for improving balance and independence in individuals aged 65 and older who had dementia and were living in nursing homes.[15] Another showed that functional training significantly improved the golf swing and fitness level of golfers aged between 60 and 80 years old.[16]

By training your muscles to work functionally, you'll prepare your body to perform well in a variety of tasks that are important to your daily life—and you can do it at home with the aid of "equipment" readily available, such as a backpack filled with canned goods, to increase the difficulty level of exercise. At most, the only exercise equipment you would need for this program is a pair of five-pound ankle weights you can easily find at Walmart or Amazon.

Exercising at Home

There are several additional benefits to exercising at home versus going to a gym:

- The ease and convenience of exercising at home removes demotivating barriers. You don't have to drive to the gym, change your clothes in a room full of strangers, or wait for workout equipment to free up.

- The gym can be an intimidating place for some older adults. But self-consciousness or fear of what others may think is not a concern with functional training at home.

- For older adults who don't function well enough to leave home without assistance, going to the gym can be difficult or impossible. Exercising at home is the only way for these people to improve strength, balance, and function.

- The price tag of a gym membership can be an obstacle for many older adults on fixed incomes. Cost is not an issue with workouts at home that require little or no equipment.

Combination Approach

The real secret to this program is the integration of higher-intensity training (discussed in the last chapter) and functional training, adapted for older adults. You won't find this combined approach to exercise for older adults in many other places, but it's a method that will allow you to safely and quickly achieve great results at home with little or no equipment.

You may be wondering at this stage why you couldn't just do something else that needs no equipment—such as walking—for exercise. It's certainly true that walking is another form of functional training that doesn't require equipment and can be good for your health, but in the next chapter I'll explain why walking alone isn't enough to reverse age-related muscle loss.

Action Steps

- To prepare yourself for exercising at home, you might like to have on hand the following items:

  - A backpack filled with heavy items (such as canned goods) for resistance.

  - A pair of adjustable ankle weights. Ideally, you'll have two ankle weights (five pounds per ankle) that you can add and subtract weights by one pound increments.

5. Walking Is Not the Best Form of Exercise

In 1989, a landmark study completed by the Cooper Institute linked daily walking to improved health.[17] The study followed 13,000 people for over eight years, and the results convinced scientists that walking could provide most of the health benefits of more conventional exercise.

This study initially gave walking a good reputation as a form of exercise; the US surgeon general even issued guidelines that encouraged Americans to walk more. Before long, walking became the exercise of choice for many Americans and has been touted as the "best exercise" by healthcare and fitness authorities. That reputation is perpetuated to this day. However, as time has progressed, more details have emerged about the effectiveness of walking as a form of exercise.

According to Dr. Paul Williams, an exercise scientist at Lawrence Berkeley Laboratory in California, Americans have been given a false sense that a stroll through the neighborhood is all they need to stay healthy.

Yet, walking as you normally would isn't intense enough. The American College of Sports Medicine recommends at least 150 minutes of moderate-intensity physical activity per week to maintain health.[18] This means working hard enough that your breathing quickens, your heart rate raises, and you break a sweat, yet you're still able to carry on a conversation.[19] In one study in Mortality and Morbidity Weekly Review, only 60 percent of adults who reported walking as their main form of exercise met these guidelines.[20] Clearly, simply walking throughout the day as you normally would is not enough.

Doesn't Reverse Age-related Muscle Loss

But even if you do meet or exceed these minimum requirements to experience the full health benefits of walking, I have some bad news: walking as a form of exercise is not enough by itself to reverse age-related muscle loss. In order to effectively reverse age-related muscle loss, you would need to do strengthening exercises. To build muscle and strength, you need to take your joints through a full range of motion with enough resistance until muscle fatigue sets in. Walking doesn't accomplish this, and there's more bad news: a lot of what you get instead is negative impact on the joints within a very limited range of movement.

Can Actually Be More Harmful

Too much walking may actually be more harmful than helpful for some older adults due to the impact and stress on the body, which can lead to wear and tear, injury, and pain.

Walking can also be dangerous for adults who are very old or weak because they could easily fall. Falls are the leading cause of death from injury in older adults, and they result from a combination of age-related changes: the natural loss of 1–2 percent of muscle mass every year from age 50—which, as we have seen, walking will not reverse—and a weaker sense of balance, declining eyesight, and side effects of medication. All of these issues together can make walking a hazard for older adults who have not developed a foundation of lower-body strength.

In summary, walking is a good exercise but is not enough by itself. It should be combined with a strengthening program like the one in this book to keep you healthy and strong.

Action Steps

- Consider the following questions:
  - What was your opinion about walking as exercise before reading this chapter?

- Where do you think your ideas about walking as exercise came from?

- How has your opinion about walking as exercise changed after reading this chapter?

In part 1, you've seen how a few minutes of simple strengthening exercises every day can enhance health and function in older adults, and provide protection against natural aging-related muscle loss. Specifically, you've learned how higher-intensity functional exercises can help you achieve great results at home with little or no workout equipment in just a couple of weeks. The best part is that it doesn't matter if you're 60 or 100 years old, if you've been active or inactive, or if your health is perfect or imperfect. It's not too late to build muscle, cultivate strength, and change your life.

Part 2:
Seven Strategies for Unlocking Your Fitness Potential

In this part of the book, I'll share seven strategies for unlocking your fitness potential. If you follow each one exactly, I guarantee you will experience dramatic improvements in your strength, balance, and energy in as little as 15 days.

What you're about to learn is distilled from my experience working one-on-one with thousands of older adults.

Part 2 Topics:

- Prioritize your hips and legs.

- Dial up the intensity, dial down the time.

- Push until you feel tired—and then push a little more.

- Take baby steps in making exercise more challenging.

- Exercise daily for the first two weeks to kickstart change.

- Distinguish between "good pain" and "bad pain."

- Eat high-quality protein to boost strength gains.

6. Prioritize Your Hips and Legs

The first strategy to unlocking your fitness potential is to prioritize your hip and leg muscles. To achieve this, I recommend exclusively working on your lower body and holding off on your upper body for the first eight weeks.

There are two important reasons why I make this recommendation for older adults. First and foremost, healthy, strong hips and legs allow you to stand and walk safely and hence be self-sufficient. While having a weak upper body can be inconvenient, weakness in your lower body negatively impacts your overall quality of life more. Developing a strong lower body with the exercises I'll show you later in this book will help you navigate your environment safely. You'll be able to remain steady on your feet even in challenging circumstances, like walking on a slippery surface; and if you do happen to fall, you're more likely to emerge unscathed if you have strong hips and legs.

Second, the muscles in your hips and legs are the largest and strongest in your entire body. Research shows that higher-intensity strength exercises targeting these muscles increase your body's production of testosterone and human growth hormones.[21] Levels of these hormones decline as we age; being able to naturally increase their production through exercise offers a wealth of benefits for older adults.[22] These include building lean muscle, increasing bone density, reducing body fat, boosting energy, and strengthening the immune system.[23]

Exclusively working your lower body and holding off on your upper body for the first eight weeks will allow you to focus on what's most important, get comfortable with the workout program, and reap a lot of gains.

That's strategy number one. Let's move on to the second strategy, which is to dial up the intensity and dial down the time on exercise.

Action Steps

- Notice whether you feel resistant to the idea of not exercising your upper body in the beginning. If so, where do you think this resistance comes from? What would help you to entertain the ideas in this chapter?

7. Dial Up the Intensity, Dial Down the Time

The second strategy to unlocking your fitness potential is to dial up the intensity, dial down the time on exercise. In chapter 3, we looked at research confirming higher-intensity exercise is safe and more effective than traditional exercise for older adults, despite its substantially lower time commitment. But the benefits of dialing up the intensity and dialing down the time don't end there; research also shows that multiple short bouts (six minutes or less) of higher-intensity exercise spread throughout the day are more effective than a single longer bout of exercise.[24]

This means you get better results from exercising for 6 minutes twice daily than from 12 minutes once daily. The total time commitment is the same for both routines, but the multiple short bouts of exercise are more effective, probably because you're able to maintain a higher intensity during your workout.

Studies also show that, given the choice between working at a higher intensity for a shorter period of time or working at a lower intensity for longer, older adults more likely will be consistent with the former than the latter.[25] Being consistent with exercise is one of the most important things you need to do to get results. It's also one of the hardest. So having an exercise program that older adults more likely will stick with, despite the increased difficulty, is critical.

There's an added benefit to these short periods of activity: it's been my experience that shorter bouts of higher-intensity exercise result in less wear and tear on the body. Higher-intensity programs require fewer repetitions of movements to achieve similar benefits compared with lower-intensity programs. This means you reduce the wear and tear effects on your body, which decreases the risk of overuse, injury, and pain.

You have seen the many reasons why dialing up the intensity, dialing down the time on exercise is ideal for older adults.

Action Steps

- Has being consistent with exercise been a challenge for you in the past? If so, do you think you would be more consistent if the exercise was at a higher intensity but for a much shorter period of time?

8. Push Until You Feel Tired—Then Push a Little More

The third strategy to unlocking your fitness potential is to push until you feel tired, and then push a little more. In the field of exercise science, this is the principle of overload. It states that a greater than normal stress on the body is required for training adaptation to take place.[26] In plain language, this means you must challenge your body to go beyond what is familiar and comfortable for improvements to take place.

While exercising, you naturally want to stop and rest or catch your breath when you start feeling tired. Your body doesn't like to do more work than it has to, and it will let you know by making you feel sore, exhausted, and consumed with the desire to quit. But if you give in to your body's demands too early and stop exercising, you won't make much progress because you're not giving your body the increased stress it needs to change.

When you continue to exercise beyond the point where you would normally quit, you signal to your body that the demands you're placing on it are the new normal. As a result, your body will very quickly change to meet these demands; this change translates directly into rapid increases in strength and endurance. Now you may be thinking that six minutes is too short of a time to push yourself past the point where you would normally quit. I assure you, it's not. Remember, our goal here is to work harder, not longer. In other words, we improve our body by increasing the intensity of exercise, not the time. For example, a person can walk a mile in 30 minutes, or they can attempt to run the same distance in 6 minutes. Although the distance is the same, the 6-minute mile pace is more intense and will yield significantly more improvements in the body than the 30-minute mile pace. At the 6-minute mile pace, most people, not just older adults, would tire and quit in less than 3 minutes. Even so, those 3 minutes of intense activity will create more improvements in endurance than walking the entire mile in 30 minutes. Let me be clear. Nowhere in this book am I going to ask you to go out and run a mile, but I hope this example clarifies that by increasing the intensity of exercise, 6 minutes is plenty of time to create massive improvements in strength and function.

80/20 Percent Technique

To push yourself, then push a little more, your goal of the first 80 percent of the workout is just to get you to the point of fatigue. Exercise during this part of the workout doesn't change your body much because you're not yet pushing your limits. Your body can handle this level of exercise quite comfortably and so does not need to change to accommodate it.

The goal of the remaining 20 percent of the workout—when you've reached your perceived limit of fatigue—is to make dramatic improvements. In this critical period near the end of your workout, when you're feeling sore, exhausted, and wanting to quit, don't. Instead, push for a few more seconds or a few more repetitions (a repetition is the number of times you perform a particular movement in your workout). In other words, you push until you feel tired—and then push a little more.

This is how you provide the greater than normal stress your body requires for training adaptations to take place. This is how you challenge your body to go beyond what is familiar and comfortable and make improvements.

You may have noticed I used the phrase "perceived limit of fatigue." Your mind will tell you to stop well before your body has reached its actual limit of fatigue because the mind doesn't like unfamiliar or uncomfortable situations. Not only is it normal to feel sore, exhausted, and consumed with the desire to quit during exercise, it's actually desirable. See it as a sign that you're doing something right.

When you push until you feel tired and then push a little more, your body will very rapidly change in ways that will surprise you and everyone who knows you.

Action Steps

- Imagine that you've reached your perceived limit of fatigue during exercise. Think about how you can get yourself to push for a few more seconds or a few more repetitions of exercise. Would it be a thought, an image, a memory, something you say out loud, or something else?

9. Take Baby Steps to Make Exercise More Challenging

The fourth strategy to unlocking your fitness potential is to take baby steps in making exercise more challenging. In the field of exercise science, this is the principle of progression. It states that a systematic increase in the workload over a period of time will result in improvements in fitness without risk of injury.[27] In other words, your body will continue to get stronger while avoiding injuries if you increase the challenge gradually.

You'll notice that the exact same workout routine will begin to feel easier over a period of days or weeks, depending on how hard you push yourself. You should be proud of this: it's a sign that your body has adapted to exercise. But once your body has adapted, you won't experience much more improvement if you continue to perform the same workout exactly as before. For your body to continually increase its strength and endurance, you have to make your routine more challenging. You can achieve this by adding a new exercise, increasing the repetitions, upping the pace, or decreasing the rest time during exercise.

I recommend taking baby steps toward making exercise more challenging. For example, you might increase the number of repetitions for a particular exercise from 10 to 12 or decrease the rest time from 30 seconds to 25. At first, you'll notice that these changes will make exercise feel more difficult. But with consistent effort over a few days or weeks, your body will adapt and exercise will feel easier again. Your goal is to repeat this process of making your exercise more challenging every time you feel your workout has become easier. By doing this in baby steps, your body will continue to get stronger and avoid injuries at the same time.

Of course, injury can result if you increase the challenge too steeply. For example, if performing 5 repetitions of exercise is difficult for you, jumping to 15 repetitions the next day would be attempting too much, too soon.

Instead, you should consider taking a baby step from 5 repetitions to 6 repetitions and sticking with this until it starts to feel easier before taking another step to seven or eight repetitions.

To avoid injuries, it's important to take baby steps and to spend a day or two and, sometimes even a week or more, with the more challenging workout to ensure that your body has fully adapted to it.

It's important to mention that taking a day or two off every week is also important to help your body adapt to exercise. However, it's been my experience that working daily for the first two weeks of this program is a powerful way to kickstart change without increasing the risk of injury.

Action Steps

- Think about whether you tend to increase the challenge of exercise too much or not enough. How would you recognize when this is happening? What can you do to find a better balance?

10. Exercise Daily for the First Two Weeks to Kickstart Change

The fifth strategy to unlocking your fitness potential is to kickstart change by exercising daily for the first two weeks. This goes against the conventional wisdom that says you should ease into a new exercise program, particularly if you've been sedentary for a while.

My experience working with literally thousands of older adults over the years tells a different story: by exercising daily for the first two weeks, your body gets the kickstart it needs to change with no added risk of injury. Unless you introduce a greater volume of exercise at the beginning of the program, your body may get stuck in low gear, and then you run the risk of seeing little to no progress for all your hard work.

To illustrate this point, I like to use the analogy of launching a rocket into space. The rocket needs a lot more energy at the beginning of the flight to overcome the inertia of Earth's gravitational force, but once it's in orbit, the amount of energy required to stay up there is minimal. Like a rocket heading for space, your body needs more effort at the start of its journey to overcome its current state of inertia.

After exercising daily for the first two weeks, you won't need to invest as much energy to continue progressing. At this stage, you can rest for one day a week. This day of rest will help your body recover and avoid injuries, and keep you motivated so you can push yourself when it's time to exercise again.

After eight weeks of exercise, you can rest for two or three days a week if you're happy with your progress, don't see a need for more gains, and just want to maintain the gains you've already made.

By following this strategy, you'll see your strength, balance, and energy launch like a rocket to new levels that'll amaze you and everyone you know.

Action Steps

- Consider how the suggestion of exercising daily for the first two weeks sits with you. Do you like it, not like it, or feel neutral about it? If you have strong feelings about it, what do you think is behind them?

11. Distinguish Between "Good Pain" and "Bad Pain"

We've all heard the saying "no pain, no gain," and it's true that physical discomfort is a part of exercise. But there is such a thing as "bad pain." The sixth strategy to unlocking your fitness potential is to make the distinction between "good pain" and "bad pain." It's important to understand this distinction so you'll know when it's safe to keep pushing yourself and when you should stop.

So what exactly is the difference between good pain and bad pain? Simply put, good pain leads to gains, while bad pain doesn't.

Good pain is a normal—and even desired—part of exercise because it's a sign that you're pushing your body hard enough to cause change. During a workout, good pain feels like soreness, burning, or fatigue in your muscles. You may also notice yourself breathing harder than normal. The human body generally dislikes being out of its comfort zone; when you experience this kind of pain, consider it a sign that you're doing something right. For better or for worse, good pain is part of the process of getting fitter.

On the other hand, bad pain indicates something might be off and that you could be working against yourself. During a workout, bad pain may be a sharp, stabbing, or shooting pain that spreads; repeated painful pops; or pain with swelling. A good rule of thumb is that if the bad pain is a one-off and you don't feel it again, it's nothing to stress about. However, if it continues to be felt when you move a particular muscle or joint, stop performing the exercise.

The line between good pain and bad pain can get a little blurred in older adults. If you're out of shape or have been sedentary for a while, it's normal to feel stiffness or aching in your body and a burning sensation in your lungs as your body gets used to working and breathing harder. It's also common to feel stiffness and aching in the lower back, hips, and knees as we age. One reason for this is age-related muscle loss, combined with the relentless force of gravity over decades, leads to painful pressure on our joints. Doctors frequently give a diagnosis of osteoarthritis for this type of pain. Fortunately, exercise has been shown to reduce pain and improve function in people with osteoarthritis in the back, hips, and knees.[28]

Many people worry about clicking or grinding in their shoulders, knees, or other joints during exercise. These "noises" are not necessarily worrisome unless they are painful. If you're really out of shape, it's also normal to feel weak and tired for a few hours after exercising; this feeling may sometimes last for an entire day. Muscle soreness often sets in six to eight hours after your exercise, and it may last for two or three days. That's normal, too.

I hope what you've learned in this chapter makes the distinction between good pain and bad pain clearer. Remember, good pain leads to gains while bad pain doesn't. By making the distinction between the two, you'll know when to keep pushing yourself during exercise and when to stop.

Action Steps

- The next time you perform physical activity that is more vigorous than normal, notice whether what you're feeling is good pain or bad pain.

- If you have stiffness or aching in your body, notice what happens after you've been inactive for a while and then start moving again. Osteoarthritis usually feels better after your body gets moving.

12. Eat High-Quality Protein to Boost Strength Gains

The seventh and final strategy to unlocking your fitness potential is to eat high-quality proteins during each meal to boost strength gains. Protein from your diet is the raw material for building muscle mass and strength.

The importance of eating enough high-quality protein cannot be overemphasized. Performing strength exercises with insufficient protein intake hinders the development of muscles.

Research shows that it's harder to reverse age-related muscle loss and improve strength in older adults if they don't have adequate protein intake.[29] Studies have also shown that older adults need more protein than their younger counterparts. Inadequate protein intake is a concern for older adults and not only contributes to muscle loss, but also results in increased skin fragility, decreased immune system function, poorer healing, and longer recuperation times after illness.[30] A review published in Current Opinion in Clinical Nutrition and Metabolic Care recommended older adults consume 25–30 grams of high-quality protein per meal to enhance muscle growth and prevent age-related muscle loss.[31]

What makes protein "high-quality"? It's a combination of three things:[32]

1. How easily your body can break down the protein into its parts (called amino acids).

2. The actual parts that a protein will become when your body breaks it down (its amino acid profile).

3. How available the parts are to support muscle maintenance and growth.

High-quality proteins are easily broken down by your body, contain all the parts your body needs to build muscle, and are readily available for your body to use. Not all sources of protein contain all the building blocks your body needs to build muscle. For example, many vegetables contain protein, but it is of low quality.

The foods below contain high-quality proteins that provide everything your body needs. Remember, the goal is to consume 25–30 grams of protein per meal:

Animal

- Chicken breast (3 ounces): 28 grams protein

- Steak (3 ounces): 26 grams protein

- Turkey (3 ounces): 25 grams protein

- Lamb (3 ounces): 23 grams protein

- Pork (3 ounces): 22 grams protein

- Egg (large): 8 grams protein

Seafood

- Salmon (3 ounces): 22 grams protein

- Tuna (3 ounces): 22 grams protein

- Tilapia (3 ounces): 22 grams protein

- Cod (3 ounces): 20 grams protein

- Rainbow trout (3 ounces): 20 grams protein

- Shrimp (3 ounces): 20 grams protein

Dairy

- Greek yogurt (6 ounces): 18 grams protein

- Cottage cheese (4 ounces): 14 grams protein

- Regular yogurt (1 cup): 11 grams protein

- Milk (1 cup): 8 grams protein

- Mozzarella cheese (1 ounce): 7 grams protein

Vegetarian/Vegan

- Blend of pinto beans and rice (1 cup): 11 grams protein

- Blend of black beans and rice (1 cup): 8 grams protein

- Tofu (3.5 ounces): 8 grams protein

- Soy milk (1 cup): 8 grams protein

When it comes to maintaining and building muscle mass and strength, eating enough high-quality protein is just as important as performing strength exercises regularly. But before making any changes to your diet, be sure to speak to your doctor.

Action Steps

- Use the list of high-quality proteins provided in this chapter to get an idea of how much protein you're consuming at each meal. Are you eating 25–30 grams of high-quality protein each time? If not, what changes can be made?

In part 2, you've learned seven strategies for unlocking your fitness potential. If you follow each one exactly, I guarantee you will experience remarkable improvements in your strength, balance, and energy in two short weeks.

Part 3:
How to Win the "Mental Game" of Exercise

Staying motivated and being consistent with exercise is the biggest obstacle most people face on their journey to fitness. In this part of the book, I'll show you how to win that mental game. I'll teach you how to develop a winning mindset that will help you overcome these obstacles and empower you to take control of your fitness.

Part 3 Topics:

- Visualization to boost strength and function.

- Three powerful techniques to make exercise a habit.

- Getting in the zone with exercise by setting "micro-goals."

- Overcoming negativity bias to stay motivated with exercise.

13. Visualization Can Boost Strength and Function

Visualization (also called mental imagery) as a technique for performance enhancement has its roots in the 1984 Olympics, when Russian researchers found that Olympians who had employed visualization techniques performed better than those who didn't.[33] Since then, visualization has been widely studied as a way of conditioning the brain for successful outcomes.

Visualization Benefits

Early studies focused mainly on performance enhancement for athletes, and scientists have now reached a consensus that mental imagery is effective for athletes of all disciplines and levels of experience, from bodybuilders to gymnasts and from novices to experts. One study published in The Sport Psychologist showed that just five minutes of visual mental practice resulted in significant improvements in overall performance for both experienced as well as novice gymnasts.[34] Another found that people who visualized strength training workouts increased their strength by 13.5 percent.[35] By simply thinking about exercise, this group made almost half the gains seen by the group that actually exercised!

The power of visualization or mental imagery isn't just for athletes. Over the last two decades, much work has been done demonstrating the effectiveness of mental practice for retraining function in older adults and people with physical disabilities like chronic pain, stroke, Parkinson's disease, and spinal cord injuries.[36] One study showed that people aged 65–85 improved their performance on an indoor obstacle course with just a single session of mental imagery training.[37]

How is visualization such a powerful tool? Here's what happens: when you visualize or imagine successful performance, you actually stimulate the same parts of the brain as when you physically perform that action.[38] Additionally, visualizing successful performance can improve confidence, which can positively impact actual performance. One study demonstrated that mental imagery improved the confidence (related to feeling "psyched up" or energized) of participants during strength training, and this was associated with a higher performance during exercise.[39]

With this in mind, I recommend that you visualize successful performance of physical activities for five minutes a day. I've found the best time to do this is while you're lying in bed before sleeping at night or after waking up in the morning. Don't worry that you haven't learned the actual exercises in this book yet. For now, you can just visualize yourself performing any physical activities you enjoy.

Guided Visualization Script

Listening to this script may be helpful. You could record yourself reading it out loud, then play back the recording when you practice visualization. You can also get an audio recording of the guided visualization script included in the free bonus resources by going here: www.sixminutefitness.com/bonus

Get into a comfortable position, away from any distractions. Close your eyes and bring your awareness to your breath. Take about a minute to breathe a little deeper and a little slower than you normally would.

Trace the movement of the breath through your body. Follow it all the way to your belly and back up, releasing any worries, stress, or tension you may feel. With each breath, relax a little deeper.

As you continue to relax and breathe, imagine yourself physically active and doing something you love, as though you were watching yourself on a movie screen. This can be an activity from the past or present.

Notice whether you're indoors or outdoors, by yourself or with others. See your entire body move with grace and ease and also notice the expression on your face. Is it one of joy? Determination? Focus?

Now shift your perspective by stepping into the image of yourself on that movie screen so that you're now entirely inside your body looking out.

Notice what it feels like to be moving freely with an abundance of energy. Give yourself permission to dream, to push beyond any boundaries or limitations. What are the sensations, feelings, and emotions that are present and alive for you as you do this?

Imagine that a dial, like the volume knob on a stereo system, appears in front of you. Turn the dial up a little and notice how it increases the brightness of your surroundings and how your positive sensations and feelings intensify along with it.

Turn that dial all the way up and notice how it also makes your body stronger, boosts your energy, and leaves you radiating with the most incredible sensations and feelings.

Now imagine that you're surrounded by the most important people from your past, present, and future. Imagine them cheering for you and encouraging you on your journey toward health, wellness, and improved physical function.

Open your hands and your heart to receive their love, joy, and encouragement. Deeply feel what it's like for your body to receive this gift.

Bring your attention back to your breath.

As you breathe, know that you can take with you the gifts you've just received. When you're ready, wiggle your fingers and toes, open your eyes, and bring yourself back to the present.

Don't worry if you find visualization difficult at first. With practice, you can visualize with more vividness and detail.

Visualization is a powerful tool for boosting strength and function even without exercising. Start today and commit to sticking with it for five minutes daily.

In the next chapter, I'll show you how to make exercise a habit with three powerful techniques.

Action Steps

- Record yourself reading the guided visualization script so you can play it back to yourself. You can also get the five-minute guided visualization recording included in the free bonus resources here: http://www.sixminutefitness.com/bonus

- Spend five minutes daily listening to the guided visualization while you're in bed before sleeping or in the morning after waking up. Start today and notice any changes physically, emotionally, and mentally over the next week.

14. Three Powerful Techniques to Make Exercise a Habit

For most people, being consistent with an exercise program is challenging. Even though you know you should exercise and you need exercise, it's not always easy to get yourself to do it. Common complaints I hear from older adults are "I don't like to exercise because it doesn't feel comfortable" or "I feel too tired to exercise." Getting fit and staying fit is not a comfortable endeavor—remember that "good pain" we talked about?—and it can be difficult to be consistent with a program when you're feeling tired.

So how do we get ourselves to exercise consistently even when we're feeling tired and would rather relax than break a sweat? The answer is to make exercise a habit—a routine of behavior that is repeated regularly and tends to occur without much thinking. In other words, something that you do almost automatically.

Research shows that it takes on average two months to form a habit.[40] The fact that it takes this length of time makes forming a habit more easily said than done because we're now dealing with the chicken-and-egg problem: you have to exercise consistently for two months to make it a habit, but it's difficult to exercise consistently unless it's already a habit. Which comes first?

Luckily, you don't have to solve this problem because the three techniques I'm about to show you will make exercise a habit in a snap.

Technique 1: Habit Stacking

One of the easiest ways to build a new habit is with a technique called habit stacking, which is the idea of attaching a habit you want to acquire to a habit you already have.[41]

This works because the old habit is already built into your brain. By mentally linking the old habit with the new habit of exercise, the old habit becomes a trigger that reminds you it's time to exercise.

The formula for habit stacking is simple: before/after <existing habit>, I will <new habit>. Print this statement out in big letters and post it in prominent places throughout your house. For example, you can make signs using the statement "Before breakfast and lunch, I will exercise," and place it in obvious spots in the bedroom, restroom, living room, and kitchen. The trick to making habit stacking work is to have these multiple reminders in places where you can easily see them.

While you can stack your new habit of exercise with any current habit that you perform daily, I've found that stacking exercise with meals works great; you'll be exercising twice daily and most people have at least two meals a day. It can be before breakfast and lunch, before lunch and dinner, or before breakfast and dinner. It doesn't matter which meals you combine with exercise, so choose what works best for you.

The purpose of habit stacking is to remind you to exercise. But if we stopped here, few people would actually take action and start exercising when they're supposed to. The second technique is designed to help you overcome this obstacle.

Technique 2: Conditioned Cues

While habit stacking will remind you when to exercise, conditioned cues will help you take action. Conditioned cues are triggers that flip a switch in your head to "go"—in this case, to begin your workout.[42]

The cues are unique to each person; experiment to discover what works best for you. It could be a specific song, the smell of fresh ground coffee beans, the sensation of cold water splashing on your face, or anything else you can think of that gets you pumped up and energized to exercise. Personally, I've found that the trick to making conditioned cues work, besides being something that gets you psyched up, is to use something that you have to physically do when it's time for exercise. For example, it's better to push a button on an electronic device to turn on a song that gets you pumped up than to set an alarm that turns the song on automatically. It's even better if you have to get up from your chair, go to the kitchen sink, and splash cold water on your face because now you're taking even more action. Remember, conditioned cues are triggers that flip a switch in your head to "go" and begin your workout. The idea is that the more action you take as part of your conditioned cue, the more likely you'll begin to exercise. To remind yourself to perform your conditioned cue, write down the action you will take below your habit stacking statement on the signs you've made.

Even after you've taken action and launched your conditioned cue, you may still feel a lack of motivation to exercise. The third technique is designed to get you over this final hurdle.

Technique 3: Intrinsic Reward Statements

Psychologists have found that intrinsic rewards, such as the sense of accomplishment we feel from achieving a personal goal, are more powerful motivators than external rewards like money, power, fame, or avoiding consequences.[43]

Thus, reminding yourself of the intrinsic rewards you get from exercise will boost your motivation when it's time to work out. The key to intrinsic rewards is to notice what is internally rewarding when you have great workouts and create a "reward statement" that makes the connection between these two things. For example, you might notice that you feel really tired and sluggish before exercise but energized and clear-headed afterward, or that you tend to feel unmotivated when it's time to exercise but pumped up once you get started. These positive changes are the building blocks of your reward statement.

It may take a bit of experimentation to pinpoint exactly what makes exercise an agreeable experience for you and to create a positive statement based on it. Here are some examples of intrinsic reward statements:

- My mind feels energized and my body feels relaxed after exercise.

- I love challenging my body with exercise to see what I can achieve.

- Once I get started with exercise, I feel pumped up and I don't want to stop.

After you've crafted your intrinsic reward statement, use it to motivate yourself to work out when the time comes. Do this by repeating the statement to yourself, out loud, a few times right after you've launched your conditioned cue.

You may find that simply saying these words out loud does not provide the boost needed to get you fully fired up for exercise. To get the full effect, you need to put a ton of passion into saying your statement while also getting your body involved. For example, you would stand with your chest open, chin lifted, and hands up and opened in front of you, and say with passion, "My mind feels energized and my body feels relaxed after exercise." Research shows that changing your posture in such a way boosts the testosterone level in your body, just like exercise does.[44] By putting a ton of passion into saying your intrinsic reward statement while also getting your body involved, you can actually alter your body chemistry to more closely match your state during exercise. As a result, you will be mentally, emotionally, and physically primed for exercise. To remind yourself to perform your intrinsic reward statement, write it down below your conditioned cue on the signs you've made.

You've seen in this chapter that habit stacking, conditioned cues, and intrinsic reward statements give you a powerful set of tools to form good exercise habits. In the next chapter, I'll show you how to get in the zone with exercise by setting "micro-goals."

Action Steps

- Decide which existing habit you would like to stack with exercise.

Create at least three signs with large letters using the formula: Before/after <existing habit>, I will exercise.

- Find an effective conditioned cue that will help you flip that switch to begin your workout. It could be a specific song, the smell of fresh ground coffee beans, the sensation of cold water splashing on your face, or anything else that gets you pumped up and energized to exercise. Once you've decided on your conditioned cue, write it down on the signs below your habit stacking statement.

- Think about what is internally rewarding when you have great workouts, and create a statement that makes the connection between the action and the reward. Once you've crafted your intrinsic reward statement, write it down on the signs below your conditioned cue.

- Place the signs you've created in prominent places throughout your house. Practice performing habit stacking, conditioned cues, and intrinsic reward statements in order a few times, and observe what happens mentally, emotionally, and physically.

15. Get in the Zone by Setting "Micro-Goals"

Also known as flow, the "zone" is a mental state in which a person is fully immersed in an activity. This state is associated with a feeling of energized focus, enjoyment of the activity, and a change in the sense of time.[45] Getting in the zone can make exercise feel less daunting, help the workout pass more quickly, and even turn it into something to look forward to.

So how do you get in the zone with exercise? First, it helps to know that you have a choice about where you place your thoughts during exercise and that your thought patterns can make exercise seem easier or harder. If your thoughts are in the future and focused on how much work you still have left to do, exercise will seem harder. On the other hand, if your thoughts are in the present and focused on the process of your workout as it unfolds, it will seem easier.

Once you know this choice exists, you can choose to keep your thoughts in the present by setting micro-goals. Micro-goals are exactly as they sound: smaller goals within bigger goals.

Endurance athletes, like marathon runners, use micro-goals all the time, whether they know it or not. Running a 26-mile marathon while thinking "I've still got 20 miles to go" can have a detrimental effect on performance because the mind is in the future. To stay in the present, marathon runners frequently set micro-goals by dividing the race into six smaller races that are each four miles long, with a two-mile bonus round at the end, for example. These smaller goals are much easier for the mind to digest, and they help the runner get in the zone during a race.

You may not be a marathon runner, but you can also set micro-goals to get in the zone during exercise. For example, the idea of performing 15 repetitions of an exercise would be harder for your mind to digest than performing 5 repetitions three times. You could break the 5 repetitions down even further by doing an "easy three" and a "quick two" and repeating that three times.

How much easier does that sound than counting straight to 15 repetitions?

There's no rule for how to break exercise down into smaller chunks. Find what works for you, and then focus solely on making it to that smaller goal. Then set another one. Then another.

Set micro-goals during exercise to keep your thoughts present and focused on the process of your workout as it unfolds. By doing this, you'll get in the zone, and exercise will seem easier and go by quicker.

In the next chapter, I'll show you how to overcome negative bias to stay motivated with exercise.

Action Steps

- Experiment with micro-goals by performing a simple exercise, such as bending and straightening your elbows. Try performing 15 repetitions of this exercise by counting straight to 15. Next, try counting an "easy three" and a "quick two" and repeating that set three times. Although you performed a total of 15 repetitions both times, you may notice that setting micro-goals made exercise seem easier and go by faster.

16. Overcome Negative Bias and Stay Motivated

As humans, we tend to pay more attention to negative experiences than to positive or neutral ones. We often focus on the negative things even when they're insignificant or inconsequential, making them seem much more important than they really are.[46] Psychologists refer to this as "negative bias," and it can have a powerful effect on our thoughts, feelings, and behaviors.

One theory on why humans concentrate on the bad things and overlook the good things is that it may simply be the brain's way of keeping us safe.[47] Earlier in human history, threats from the outside world were literally a matter of life or death. Those individuals who were more attuned to danger or who paid more attention to the bad things around them were more likely to survive. However, unlike our ancestors, we no longer need to constantly be on high alert to survive, so this hard-wired tendency is not as useful as it once was. In fact, our brain's well-intentioned tendency to overemphasize the negative can be counterproductive to our goals. Fortunately, we can overcome our brain's negative bias so we can stay motivated and consistent with exercise.

How to Overcome Negative Bias

The first thing you can do to overcome negative bias is to become aware of any negative internal dialogue and replace it with positive self-talk. Start paying attention to the type of thoughts that run through your mind. If you notice negative thoughts about exercise, stop them immediately and replace them with a positive affirmation. Imagine you catch yourself thinking "I don't feel like exercising today." You can stop that thought and replace it with "I always feel great after exercise." If your brain is telling you "I'm feeling tired," you can replace that thought with "Exercise energizes me."

The key is to stop the negative self-talk as soon as you catch it and immediately replace it with positive self-talk that resonates with you.

The second thing you can do to overcome negative bias is to give extra attention to the good things that happen during exercise or as a result of exercise. Because negative experiences are more easily stored in your long-term memory, you need to make more effort to remember positive experiences. So when something good happens during or because of exercise, take a moment to really focus on it. Replay the moment several times in your mind, and notice the wonderful feelings the memory evokes. In other words, celebrate it.

For example, if you notice that you were able to push out one additional repetition of an exercise than in a previous session, celebrate it. If you notice yourself getting up from a chair more easily because you're getting stronger with exercise, take a moment to celebrate it. On the other hand, if you didn't improve, or maybe even went backward a little on your performance compared with a previous session—as sometimes happens—take note of it, and then shift your attention to one of the good results of exercise instead.

Why You Should Focus on Positive Self-Talk

Research in the workplace shows that when the ratio of positive and negative interactions is about five to one, people feel motivated to continue doing what they're doing well and do it with more vigor and determination.[48] Psychologist John Gottman found something similar in the domestic setting: the single biggest determinant of whether a relationship endures is the ratio of positive to negative comments the partners make to one another—the optimal ratio being five positive comments for every negative one.[49]

Clearly, in both work and life, positive and negative experiences have an important impact on success or failure. Imagine what we can achieve by changing our relationship with exercise from a negative to a positive one!

By replacing negative self-talk with positive self-talk and by giving extra attention to the good things that result from exercise, you will overcome your brain's negative bias so you can stay motivated and be more consistent with exercise.

Action Steps

- Pay attention to the type of thoughts that run through your mind over the next 24 hours, and keep track of how many are positive and how many are negative. Is the ratio of positive to negative self-talk anywhere close to five to one? You can do this assessment with any thoughts, not just those related to exercise.

- See what changes mentally, emotionally, and physically when you improve the ratio of positive to negative self-talk over the next 24 hours. You can do this by catching negative self-talk and replacing it with positive self-talk and by giving extra attention to good things that happen throughout your day. Apply what you learn from this to exercise.

In part 3, you've learned several important strategies for winning the mental game of exercise. In part 4, I'll show you the nuts and bolts of the six-minute workout.

Part 4:
Nuts and Bolts of the Six-Minute Workout

In this part of the book, I'll explain the nuts and bolts of the six-minute workout. After reading this section, you'll know everything there is to know about the six-minute workout and be able to perform it with precision.

Part 4 Topics:

- Personalization, precision, programming, and the "Big Three."

- Big Three Level I: for those who have difficulty standing.

- Big Three Level II: for those who have difficulty walking.

- Big Three Level III: for those who are high functioning.

- Big Three Level IV: upper body exercises after eight weeks.

17. Personalization, Precision, Programming, and the "Big Three"

So, what do I mean by the "Big Three"? The Big Three is a minimalist exercise program that focuses on three basic movements the human body is built to perform. These movements are tailored to your level of function and put together in a way that maximizes their benefit.

Wait a minute ... the entire program is only three exercises? Yes, that's what I'm telling you. And there's a good reason: research shows that humans may only be able to hold three or four things in the conscious mind at one time.[50]

My experience working with thousands of clients over the years confirms this finding. When I ask people to focus on more than three exercises on their own, the quality of movement generally goes down the drain. This can result in either time wasted on ineffective workouts in the best-case scenario, or injuries in the worst-case scenario.

But removing this mental clutter isn't the only thing that makes the Big Three work, and it goes much deeper than just performing three exercises. The program is super effective because it combines functional training and higher-intensity training adapted for older adults. You will remember that functional training is exercise that mimics activities or specific skills you perform at home, at work, or in sports to help you thrive in your daily life. You may also recall that HIIT is an approach to training that alternates between short periods of higher-intensity exercise and less intense recovery periods.

The Big Three's combination of functional training and higher-intensity training adapted for older adults stimulates the body in powerful ways to generate results fast.

The important concepts behind the Big Three are personalization, precision, and programming.

Personalization

The Big Three adapts exercise to different levels of function, physical limitations, and fitness goals common in older adults. This type of personalization makes exercise safe and effective while fulfilling the needs of most people.

The Big Three has four levels:

- Level I is designed for older adults who can't stand or have difficulty standing for at least six minutes with or without support (e.g., a walker), due to limitations in strength, balance, or energy.

- Level II is designed for older adults who have no difficulty standing but who lack the strength or energy to walk at a vigorous pace for at least six minutes. This level is also appropriate for those who have difficulty going up and down a flight of stairs.

- Level III is designed for older adults who are high functioning. This means they can walk at a vigorous pace for more than six minutes and can go up and down several flights of stairs with no difficulty.

- Level IV is designed to exercise the upper body after eight weeks of Level II or Level III exercise.

Precision

Precision refers to the quality of the exercise as performed. Also known as proper form or technique, precision considers factors like body alignment, movement angle, and range of motion, all of which are essential for successful training.

With exercise, the difference between what is precise and not precise can be as little as an inch in alignment or movement. Just one inch can make the difference between injury and no injury, and between progress and no progress.

I'm big on precision, for obvious reasons. I'll provide detailed yet simple instructions in the next few chapters to help you perform exercise with precision.

Programming

Programming refers to the design of the workout session: the number and type of exercises performed, the number of repetitions for each one, the length of rest breaks between exercises, and the order in which the exercises are performed. Programming also considers factors such as the number of times exercise is performed in a day, the time taken between exercise sessions if performed more than once daily, whether the same or different exercises are used, and how many times a week exercise is performed.

You need to consider these factors because the exact same exercises can be adapted to people with different needs—and even yield different results for the same person—depending on how the pieces are put together.

Programming for the Big Three is meant to maximize its ability to improve strength, balance, and energy safely, quickly, and effectively in adults from ages 60–100.

Here are the programming considerations for the Big Three:

- **Number of exercises:** Three.

- **Sessions a day exercise is performed:** Two times a day.

- **Time spaced between sessions:** At least three hours apart; exercises should preferably be performed before meals.

- **Days a week exercise is performed:** Exercise seven days a week for the first two weeks, with exercise reduced to six days a week after that.

- **Repetitions:** Each exercise is performed for up to 15 repetitions in sequence without rest. Whatever amount of repetitions you do should be the same for all exercises within a workout session. One round is counted every time you complete all three of the exercises. Your goal is to complete as many rounds as possible in six minutes, or until exhaustion.

- **Rest break:** Short rest breaks of up to 30 seconds are allowed, but only if you're completely exhausted and only after a full round of exercise has been completed.

- **Order of exercises:** This changes daily in a rotational manner. For example, on day one, you'll perform exercises in the order ABC, on day two CAB, and day three BCA.

- **Same or different routines:** Same set of exercises daily until you're ready for a higher level. If you're on the border between levels, you can perform the harder level for your first session and the easier one for your second session.

- **Upper body exercises:** Performed once daily after eight weeks of Level II or Level III.

Now you understand the concept behind the Big Three and how personalization, precision, and programming can bring rapid change to your body, no matter what your age or level of function.

In the next chapter, we'll get into the nuts and bolts of how to perform Big Three Level I.

Action Steps

- Read the description of each level of the Big Three, and decide which one is the best fit for you. You can go through each chapter in this part of the book to help you decide, or you can skip directly to the chapter with the level of Big Three that you feel is the best fit for you.

18. Big Three Level I

Level I is designed for older adults who can't stand or who have difficulty standing for at least six minutes with or without support, such as a walker, due to limitations in strength, balance, or energy.

All exercises for Level I are performed while lying on your back.

I don't recommend performing these exercises on the floor because getting up again may be difficult or dangerous.

You'll be ready for Level II once you can stand for six minutes without too much difficulty.

Exercise 1: Straight Leg Raise

The first exercise in Level I is the straight leg raise. This exercise primarily works the large muscles on the front of the thighs, called the quadriceps. Known as antigravity muscles, these muscles work to oppose the effects of gravity, helping you maintain an upright and balanced posture in standing. The quadriceps are important muscles that help you go from sitting to standing and maintain your body in the standing position.

Equipment

Required

- A firm surface to lie down on; a softer bed or couch will work if a firm surface is not available.

To decrease challenge (optional)

- None.

To increase challenge (optional)

- Ankle weights.

Performing the straight leg raise

Starting position

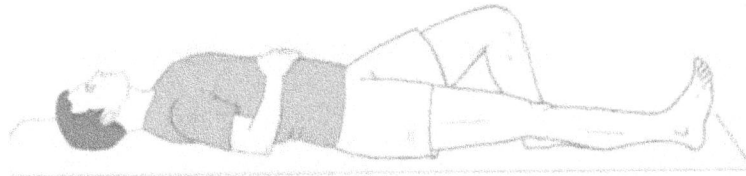

- Lie on your back with one knee straight and the other knee bent with the sole of your foot flat on the surface.

- Ensure that the toes of your straight leg are pointed straight up and not turned to either side.

- Tighten the front thigh muscles of your straight leg.

Movement to ending position

- Lift the straight leg while keeping the front thigh muscles tight, the knee straight, and the toes pointed straight up. Make sure to breathe throughout the movement.

Ending position

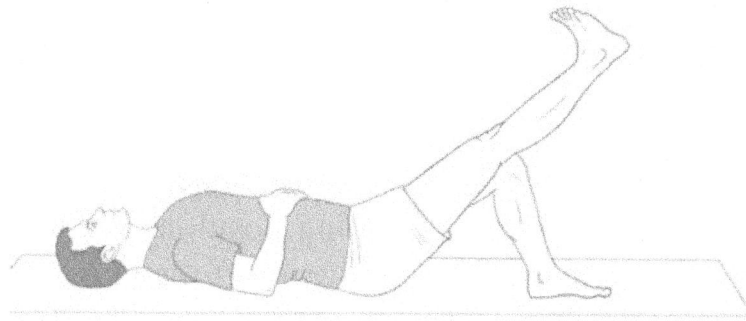

- The straight leg is lifted so that the heel is two to three feet above the surface. Hold for a half second.

Return to starting position

- Lower the leg back to the starting position with control while keeping the front of the thigh muscles tight, the knee straight, and the toes pointed straight up.

Repetitions

- Repeat the movement at a moderate pace on the same leg up to 15 times. Repeat this exercise on the opposite leg once you've completed your repetitions on one side.

Points to consider

- Make sure you're lying relatively flat while performing this exercise. The more your body is inclined, the less range of motion your leg gets, which means less work for your muscles, making the exercise less effective. You can have your head elevated on a pillow if you find that more comfortable.

- Make sure the toes of the straight leg are pointed straight up throughout this exercise. We tend to have our toes turned outward an inch or more, which can create muscle imbalances.

- Make sure the front thigh muscles of the lifting leg stay tight and the knee is straight throughout the exercise. This ensures the muscles get as much work as possible.

- Make sure the bottom of the heel is no higher than three feet from the surface when the leg is in the ending position. We tend to lift the leg too high, which actually takes the work off the muscle and reduces the effectiveness of this exercise.

To decrease challenge

- If you're not strong enough to lift your leg to the correct height, lift it to wherever you can manage right now. You'll get stronger over time.

To increase challenge

- Modify the starting position so that the heel of the straight leg is hovering a half-inch above the surface. Perform the exercise so that your heel doesn't touch the surface at any time.

- Add an ankle weight to your leg. Start by placing the weight above your knee, lowering it to your ankle as you get stronger. This helps to gradually increase the torque around your hip and knee to protect you from injury.

Exercise 2: Single-Leg Tuck

The second exercise in Level I is the single-leg tuck. Like the straight leg raise, this exercise primarily works the large antigravity muscles at the front of the thighs, but it also works the hip flexor muscles that lift your legs from the ground.

Weakness in the hip flexor muscles can make the legs feel heavy and is a common reason why older adults drag their feet when they walk; this altered gait results in a high risk for falls. Strengthening the hip flexor muscles will make your legs feel less heavy and help you pick up your feet to clear the ground.

Equipment

Required

- A firm surface to lie down on; a softer bed or couch will work if a firm surface is not available.

To decrease challenge (optional)

- None.

To increase challenge (optional)

- Ankle weights.

Performing the single-leg tuck

Starting position

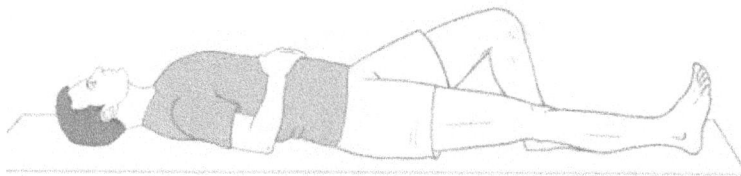

- Lie on your back with one knee straight and the other knee bent with the sole of your foot flat on the surface.
- Ensure that the toes of your straight leg are pointed straight up and not turned to either side.

Movement to ending position

- Lift the straight leg about 12 inches off the surface. Then bring the knee of the lifted leg toward your chest until the hip and the knee are both bent at a 90-degree angle. Make sure to breathe throughout the movement.

Ending position

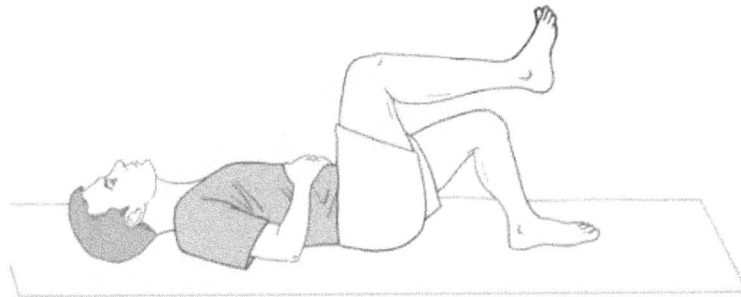

- The leg that you lifted is bent 90 degrees at the hip and knee. Hold for a half second.

Return to starting position

- Straighten the lifted leg while lowering it back to the starting position with control and ensuring that the toes are pointed straight up.

Repetitions

- Repeat the movement at a moderate pace on the same leg up to 15 times. Repeat this exercise on the opposite leg once you've completed your repetitions on one side.

Points to consider

- Make sure you're lying relatively flat while performing this exercise.

The more your body is inclined, the less range of motion your leg gets, which means less work for your muscles, making the exercise less effective. You can have your head elevated on a pillow if you find that more comfortable.

- Make sure the toes of the straight leg are pointed straight up throughout this exercise. We tend to have our toes turned outward an inch or more, which can create muscle imbalances.

- Make sure the knee does not bend too much during the movement portion of this exercise. The tendency is for the heel to drop toward the buttocks, which bends the knee too much and reduces the work on the muscles, making the exercise less effective. The movement should look like you're marching in place on one leg while lying on your back.

- In the ending position, make sure the hip and knee of the moving leg are bent 90 degrees. The body should be in the shape of a lowercase letter h, or a chair, with your lower legs making the legs of the chair, your upper leg perpendicular making the seat, and your body making the backrest. We tend to overshoot the movement so that the hip and knee are bent too much in the ending position. This is a coordination issue that will improve with practice.

To decrease challenge

- If you're not strong enough to perform this exercise with the proper form, have someone help you by placing one hand on your knee and one hand on your ankle to lightly guide you through the motion.

To increase challenge

- Modify the starting position so that the heel of the straight leg is hovering a half-inch above the surface. Perform the exercise so that your heel doesn't touch the surface at any time.

- Add an ankle weight to your leg. Start by placing the weight above your knee, lowering it to your ankle as you get stronger. This helps to gradually increase the torque around your hip and knee to protect you from injury.

Exercise 3: Hip Raise

The third exercise in Level I is the hip raise. This exercise primarily works the powerful muscles of your buttocks, commonly referred to as the glutes. The glutes are important muscles that help you go from sitting to standing and also oppose the effects of gravity to help you maintain an upright and balanced posture when standing.

Equipment

Required

- A firm surface to lie on; a softer bed or couch will work if a firm surface is not available.

To decrease challenge (optional)

- None.

To increase challenge (optional)

- Ankle weights.

Performing the hip raise

Starting position

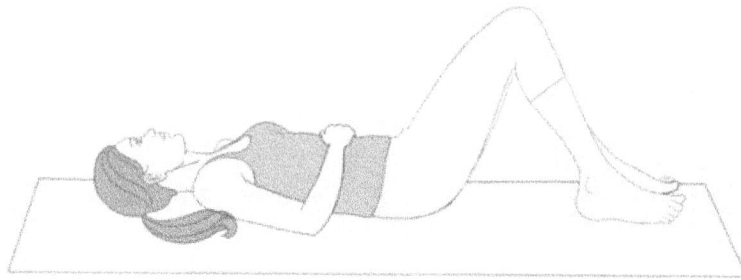

- Lie on your back with your hands folded together on your stomach, both knees bent at slightly less than 90 degrees, feet flat on the surface with toes pointed straight forward, and feet and knees about six inches apart.

- Tighten your buttocks and abdominal muscles.

Movement to ending position

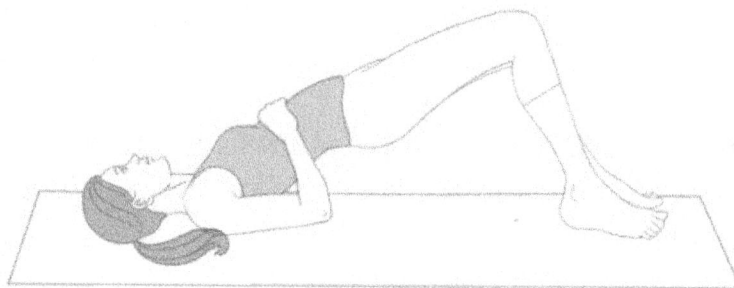

- Lift your hips up by pushing down on your feet while keeping your abdominal muscles tight. Make sure to breathe throughout the movement.

Ending position

- Your hips are lifted so that your body is in a straight line from your knees to shoulders, and your knees are bent at about 90 degrees. Hold for one to two seconds.

Return to starting position

- Lower the hips back to the starting position with control while keeping your abdominal muscles tight.

Repetitions

- Repeat the movement at a moderate pace up to 15 times.

Points to consider

- Make sure you're lying relatively flat while performing this exercise. You can have your head elevated on a pillow if you find that more comfortable.

- Make sure the toes of both feet are pointed straight forward and not turned outward or inward. Also, ensure your feet are aligned so the toes of one foot are not ahead or behind the toes of the other. This will avoid creating muscle imbalances.

- Make sure that both knees are bent to slightly less than 90 degrees in the starting position. You can accomplish this by bending your knees to 90 degrees and then sliding both heels about two inches toward your buttocks. This is so that your knees will be at a 90-degree angle when your hips are fully raised in the ending position, which optimizes the work on your glute muscles while also protecting your lower back.

- Make sure to keep the feet and knees six inches apart during this exercise. You may tend to collapse the knees inward during movement, which may place strain on your joints.

- Your hands should be resting on your stomach so you avoid the temptation of using them to assist with the movement.

To decrease challenge

- If you're not strong enough to lift your hips to the correct height, lift to wherever you can; you'll get stronger over time.

To increase challenge

- Place ankle weights on top of your pelvis to increase the resistance.

In this chapter, you learned the nuts and bolts of performing Big Three Level I. The next chapter provides detailed instructions for Big Three Level II.

Action Steps

- If this is the right level for you, spend some time going through the steps of each exercise until the movement feels natural. Try to cultivate an experimental mindset, and slow things down to learn the movements correctly. It's okay if your performance is less than perfect at first. Notice what "right" feels like in your body as you start to get the hang of each exercise.

- If you haven't done so already, get the exercise illustrations for this level, included in the free bonus resources at www.sixminutefitness.com/bonus. Post the illustrations on the wall in the room where you'll be exercising so you can see them easily.

19. Big Three Level II

This level is designed for older adults who have no difficulty standing but who lack the strength or energy to walk at a vigorous pace for at least six minutes. Level II is also designed for those who have difficulty going up and down a flight of stairs.

You'll be ready for Level III once you can walk at a vigorous pace for more than six minutes.

Exercise 1: Chair Squat

The first exercise in Level II is the chair squat. This exercise primarily works the large muscles on the front of the thighs (the quadriceps) and the powerful muscles of your buttocks, commonly referred to as the glutes. Known as antigravity muscles, they work to oppose the effects of gravity and help you maintain an upright and balanced posture when standing. Exercising these muscles helps with essential activities like standing up from the toilet, getting out of bed, and getting out of a chair. Additionally, strengthening these muscles will improve your ability to walk and climb stairs.

Equipment

Required

- A sturdy chair. The back of the chair should be against something solid like a wall, couch, or heavy table to prevent the chair from moving. The seat should be at the right height so that your knees are bent at about 90 degrees when you sit with your feet flat on the ground. You can put one or two small pillows to raise the seat if needed.

To decrease challenge (optional)

- One or two small pillows to raise the seat height.

To increase challenge (optional)

- A sturdy backpack loaded with heavy items such as weights, books, canned goods, or similar items to increase resistance.

Performing the chair squat

Starting position

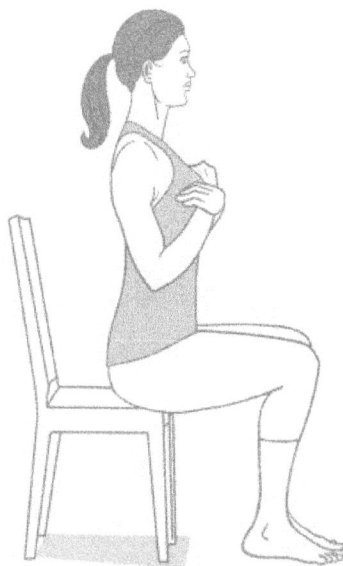

- Sit on the front half of the seat with your feet back so that the front of your feet are underneath your knees, your feet are about hip-width apart (6–12 inches), your toes are pointing forward, and your arms are crossed in front of your chest.

- Your knees should be bent to about 90 degrees in sitting with your feet touching the ground. If the seat is too low, you can adjust the height by placing pillows on the seat.

Movement to ending position

- Lean forward at the waist to bring your nose over your toes, and stand up by pushing with your legs to a full upright standing position. Make sure to breathe throughout the movement.

Ending position

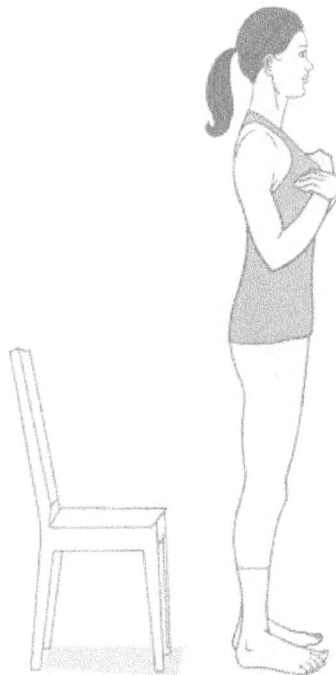

- You are standing upright with your feet about 6–12 inches apart, your toes pointing forward, and your arms crossed in front of your chest.

Return to starting position

- Lower yourself back to the starting position with control by bending at the waist to bring your nose over your toes and reaching your hips back toward the seat. Be sure to sit back down completely.

Repetitions

- Repeat the movement at a moderate pace up to 15 times.

Points to consider

- Make sure to perform this exercise without using your arms to push up on the chair; in this way, you will train your legs to do the work. Older adults with weaker legs tend to go from sitting to standing using their arms for help. This habit prevents the leg muscles from being worked on, which is why I teach this exercise with the arms crossed in front of the chest.

- Make sure your feet remain about hip-width apart (6–12 inches) with your toes pointing forward during this exercise. You may tend to move one or both feet out of this position, which can create muscle imbalances.

- Make sure the chair didn't move out of position before you sit down, as this can result in a fall and injury.

To decrease challenge

- Use one or two pillows to increase the seat height. You can remove them to gradually lower the seat as you get stronger.

- If you're still having difficulty with this exercise even with pillows on the chair, you can place your hands on your knees to help push yourself up to the standing position. Pushing off your knees is different than pushing off the chair because your legs still get all the work.

- If you're still having difficulty with this exercise even with pushing off your knees, ask someone to assist you by having them stand in front of you. Grab on to their hands with your hands, and use your arms to help pull yourself up to the standing position. Gradually reduce the amount of help you need from your arms as you get stronger.

To increase challenge

- Perform the exercise while wearing a sturdy backpack loaded with heavy items to increase the resistance.

Exercise 2: Heel Lift

The second exercise in Level II is the heel lift. This exercise primarily works the calf muscles on the back of the lower leg. These muscles are also antigravity muscles that oppose the effects of gravity to help you maintain an upright and balanced posture in standing.

Because these muscles help return circulating blood back to the heart, they are sometimes called your body's "second heart." Strong calf muscles serve better in this role to prevent or reduce swelling in the feet and to prevent blood clots from forming. Strong calf muscles are also important for daily activities, such as using the feet to push off and propel your body forward while walking, or standing on your tiptoes to reach up for something.

Equipment

Required

- A sturdy chair. The back of the chair should be against something solid like a wall, couch, or heavy table to prevent the chair from moving. You will be performing this exercise with this chair behind you for safety in case you fall backward.

- A walker or a second chair with a high backrest placed in front of the first chair for balance.

To decrease challenge (optional)

- None.

To increase challenge (optional)

- A sturdy backpack loaded with heavy items, such as weights, books, canned goods, or similar items to increase resistance.

Performing the heel lift

Starting position

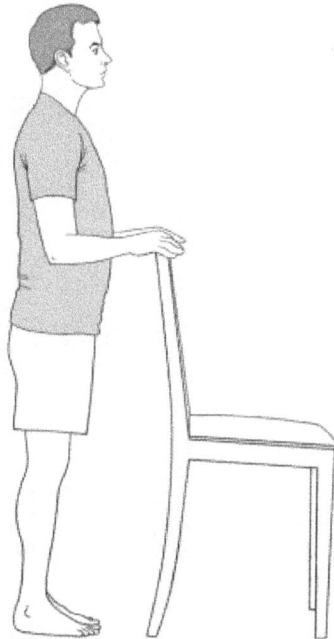

- Stand in front of the chair with your feet about hip-width apart (6–12 inches), your toes pointing forward, and your hands placed lightly on a walker or the backrest of a second chair for balance.

Movement to ending position

- With your knees straight and without leaning forward, lift your heels off the floor. Make sure to breathe throughout the movement.

Ending position

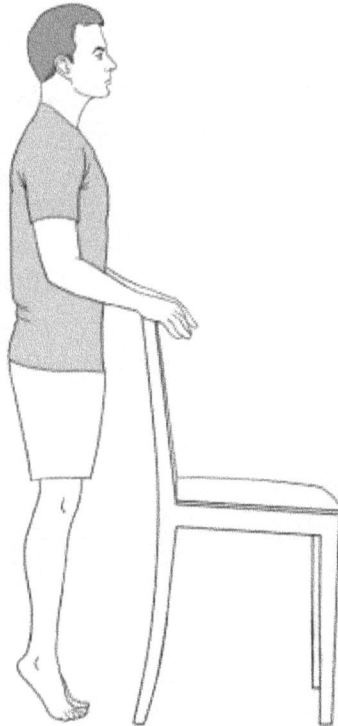

- You are on your toes with your heels lifted off the floor. Your feet remain about 6–12 inches apart with your toes pointing forward and your knees straight. Hold for a half second.

Return to starting position

- Lower your heels back to the floor with control.

Repetitions

- Repeat the movement at a moderate pace up to 15 times.

Points to consider

- You may tend to bend your knees when lifting the heels off the floor, which prevents your calf muscles from getting the work they need. So make sure to keep your knees straight throughout this exercise.

- There can also be a tendency to lean forward, which also reduces the effectiveness of the exercise. Make sure that your body is moving straight up and down throughout this exercise and that your hands are only lightly placed on the walker or the backrest of the second chair for balance.

To decrease challenge

- If you're not strong enough to lift your heels all the way up, lift them to wherever you can; you'll get stronger over time.

To increase challenge

- Perform the exercise while wearing a sturdy backpack loaded with heavy items to increase the resistance.

- Take your hands off the walker or the backrest of the second chair to work on balance. I recommend hovering the hands an inch above the support so you can quickly grab it if you lose your balance.

Exercise 3: High Knees Marching

The third exercise in Level II is high knees marching. This exercise works the large antigravity muscles on the front of the thigh and the hip flexor muscles on the front of the hip that lift your legs from the ground.

Since weakness in the hip flexor muscles can make the legs feel heavy, resulting in dragging your feet while you walk and increasing the risk for falls, you need to strengthen these muscles. Strengthening the hip flexor muscles will make the legs feel lighter and help with picking up the feet to clear the ground. This exercise will improve your ability to walk longer distances, walk up an incline or on uneven surfaces, and climb stairs.

Equipment

Required

- A sturdy chair. The back of the chair should be against something solid like a wall, couch, or heavy table to prevent the chair from moving. You will be performing this exercise with this chair behind you for safety in case you fall backward.

- A walker or a second chair with a high backrest placed in front of the first chair for balance.

To decrease challenge

- None.

To increase challenge

- Ankle weights.

Performing high knees marching

Starting position

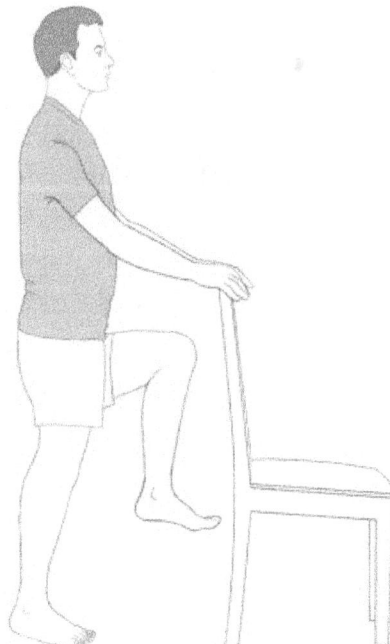

- Stand in front of the chair with your feet about hip-width apart (6–12 inches), your toes pointing forward, and your hands placed lightly on a walker or the backrest of a second chair for balance.

- Your right leg is on the ground, and your left leg is lifted with hip and knee bent 90 degrees.

- The walker or the second chair should be placed farther forward than in the heel lift, to make room for you to lift your knees.

Movement to ending position

- Lower the left leg to the ground next to the right leg, and lift the right leg up in a marching motion until the hip and knee are 90 degrees. Make sure to breathe throughout the movement.

Ending position

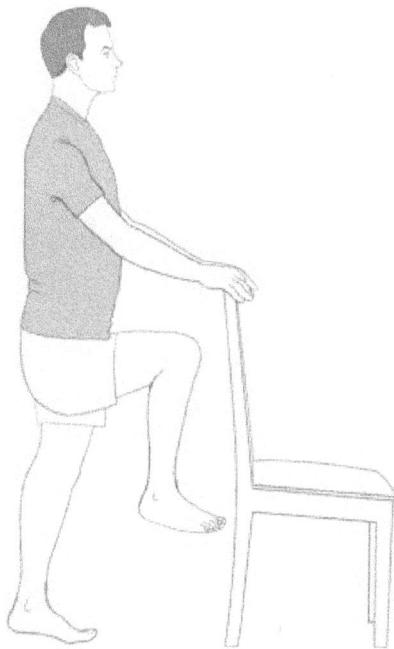

- The right leg is lifted with hip and knee bent 90 degrees. The left leg is on the ground.

Return to starting position

- Lower your right leg back to the ground, and lift your left leg back up to the starting position.

Repetitions

- Repeat the movement at a moderate pace up to 15 times on each side, taking alternating steps in place.

Points to consider

- Make sure the lifted leg's hip and knee are at 90 degrees in the ending position. The body should look like the letter h, or the shape of a chair, with your lower legs making the chair leg, your upper leg making the seat, and your body making the backrest. The tendency is to not lift the leg up high enough, which prevents your hip flexor muscles from working through most of their range of motion. The other tendency is to bend the knee too much when lifting, which prevents the hip flexors from getting the work they need.

- Make sure the support in front of you is not too close. Otherwise, you may hit your knee on it when you lift your leg.

To decrease challenge

- If you're not strong enough to lift your leg all the way up, lift it to wherever you can; you'll get stronger over time.

To increase challenge

- Perform the exercise while wearing ankle weights to increase the resistance.

- Take your hands off the walker or the second chair to work on balance. I recommend hovering the hands an inch above the support so that you can quickly grab it if you lose your balance.

In this chapter, you learned the nuts and bolts of performing Big Three Level II. The next chapter provides detailed instructions on how to perform Big Three Level III. Before proceeding, you should bear in mind that Level III is challenging; it's best to stick with Level II if you have any back, hip, or knee issues.

Action Steps

- If this is the right level for you, spend some time going through the steps of each exercise until the movement feels natural. Try to cultivate an experimental mindset, and slow things down to learn the movements correctly. It's okay if your performance is less than perfect at first. Notice what "right" feels like in your body as you start to get the hang of each exercise.

- If you haven't done so already, get the exercise illustrations for this level, included in the free bonus resources at www.sixminutefitness.com/bonus. Post the illustrations on the wall in the room where you'll be exercising so you can see them easily.

20. Big Three Level III

This level is designed for older adults who are high functioning. This means they can walk at a vigorous pace for more than six minutes and can go up and down several flights of stairs with no difficulty.

This level is challenging, so it's best to stick with Level II if you have any back, hip, or knee issues.

Exercise 1: Stationary Lunge

The first exercise in Level III is the stationary lunge. This exercise works the large quadriceps muscles on the front of the thighs and the powerful glute muscles of your buttocks. You will recall from previous levels that these are known as antigravity muscles because they work to oppose the effects of gravity, which helps you maintain an upright and balanced posture when standing.

The stationary lunge is a single-leg movement that works each side of your body independently. Single-leg movements are important because they help to correct the imbalances between the two sides of the body that exist in most people and activate your stabilizing muscles to develop balance, coordination, and stability.

Lunges are important for helping you get up from the ground, or any low surface, and are a great exercise to strengthen, sculpt, and tone your body while also improving overall fitness and enhancing athletic performance.

Equipment

Required

- None.

To decrease challenge (optional)

- A sturdy table or countertop.

To increase challenge (optional)

- A sturdy backpack loaded with heavy items such as weights, books, canned goods, or similar items to increase resistance.

Performing the stationary lunge

Starting position

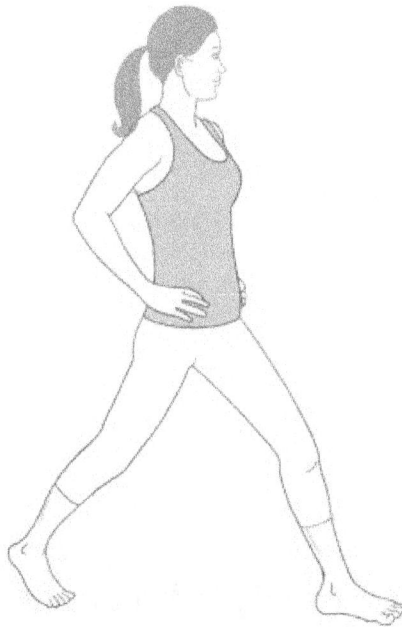

- Stand with your feet about hip-width apart (6–12 inches), your toes pointing forward, and your hands resting on your waist.

- Take a big step forward with one leg (about 2–3 feet for most people). Ensure the toes of your front foot are pointed straight forward and the heel of your back foot is lifted off the floor.

- Keep your back and upper body straight, and ensure that most of your weight is on the heel of your front foot.

Movement to ending position

- Lower your body straight down until your front knee is at about a 90-degree angle and your front thigh is parallel to the floor. Make sure to breathe throughout the movement.

Ending position

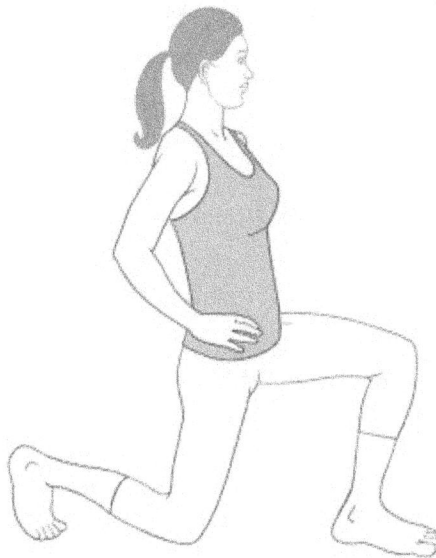

- Your front knee is bent at about a 90-degree angle directly above your front ankle, and your front thigh is parallel to the floor.

- Your back heel is lifted off the floor, and your back knee is lightly touching the floor.

Return to starting position

- Return to the starting position by pushing through the heel of your front foot.

Repetitions

- Repeat the movement at a moderate pace on the same leg up to 15 times. Repeat this exercise on the opposite leg once you've completed your repetitions on one side.

Points to consider

- To protect your front knee from injury, do not move it ahead of your front toes at any time during this exercise. If your knee does go over your toes, try lowering your body straight down during this exercise. If this doesn't resolve the issue, you may need to take a bigger step forward with the front leg.

- Additionally, do not move your front knee inward toward the midline of your body during this exercise. It should stay aligned with the second and third toes of your front foot throughout the movement.

To decrease challenge

- Stand in front of a sturdy table or countertop and place your hands on it for assistance.

To increase challenge

- Perform the exercise while wearing a sturdy backpack loaded with heavy items to increase the resistance.

Exercise 2: Step-Up

The second exercise in Level III is the step-up. This exercise also works the antigravity muscles: the quadriceps in the thighs and the powerful glute muscles of your buttocks.

The step-up is a single-leg movement in standing that works each side of your body independently and activates your stabilizing muscles to develop balance, coordination, and stability.

The step-up works the same muscles as the stationary lunge, but at a different angle; this provides different benefits. While lunges will help you get up from the ground, or any low surface, step-ups will help you lift your body up a stair, incline, or any high surface. Step-ups are a great exercise to strengthen, sculpt, and tone your body while also improving overall fitness and enhancing athletic performance.

Equipment

Required

- A step (8–24 inches).

To decrease challenge (optional)

- A lower step (8–12 inches), like a single step in a staircase.

To increase challenge (optional)

- A higher step (12–24 inches), like a sturdy chair.
- A sturdy backpack loaded with heavy items such as weights, books, canned goods, or similar items to increase resistance.

Performing the step-up

Starting position

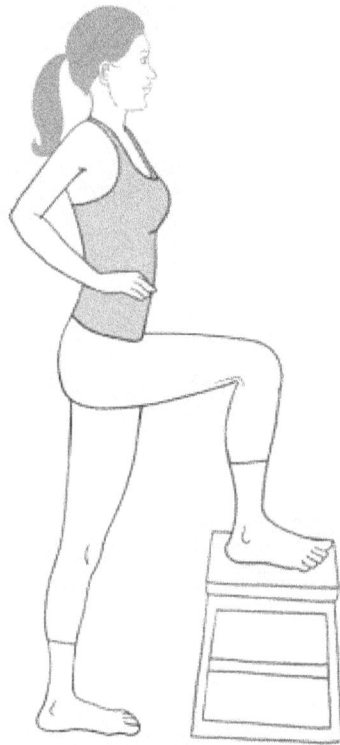

- Stand with one foot on the step and the other foot on the ground below the step.

- Make sure your feet are about hip-width apart (6–12 inches), your toes are pointing straight forward, and your hands are resting on your waist.

Movement to ending position

- Lift your body up the step by pressing through the front foot until that leg is straight.

- At the same time, lift your opposite leg up until the knee is about waist level. Make sure to breathe throughout the movement.

Ending position

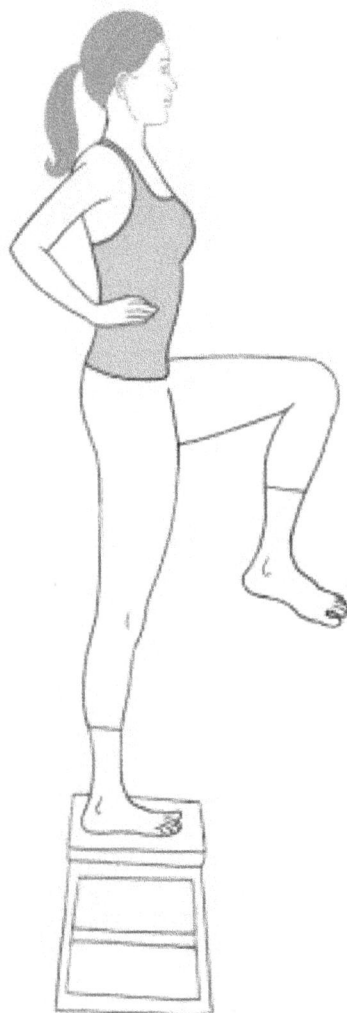

- The leg that is on the step is straight, and the leg that is lifted is bent to about 90 degrees at the hips and knees.

Return to starting position

- Lower your body back to the starting position by bringing the leg that is lifted back down to the ground and bending the knee of the leg that is on the step.

Repetitions

- Repeat the movement at a moderate pace on the same leg up to 15 times. Repeat this exercise on the opposite leg once you've completed your repetitions on one side.

Points to consider

- To protect your front knee from injury, do not move it ahead of your front toes at any time during this exercise. If your knee does go in front of your toes, try keeping your body straight, and avoid leaning too far forward as you lift your body during this exercise.

- Additionally, do not move your front knee inward toward the midline of your body during this exercise. It should stay aligned with the second and third toes of your front foot throughout the movement.

To decrease challenge

- Use a lower step (8–12 inches), like a single step in a staircase. Gradually work your way up to a higher step as you get stronger.

- Place one hand on a wall or a rail for balance.

To increase challenge

- Use a higher step (12–24 inches), like a sturdy chair.

- Perform the exercise while wearing a sturdy backpack loaded with heavy items to increase the resistance.

Exercise 3: Single-Leg Heel Lift

The third exercise in Level III is the single-leg heel lift. This exercise primarily works the muscles on the back of the lower leg called the calf muscles. Like the quadriceps and glutes, these muscles are also antigravity muscles that help you maintain an upright and balanced posture when standing.

Because they help to return circulating blood back to the heart, the calf muscles are sometimes called your body's "second heart." Strong calf muscles serve better in this role to prevent or reduce swelling in the feet and also prevent blood clots from forming. Strong calf muscles are also important for daily activities, such as using the feet to push off and propel your body forward while walking, or standing on your tiptoes to reach for something.

Equipment

Required

- A step.

- A wall or rail that you can place your hands on for balance.

To decrease challenge (optional)

- None.

To increase challenge (optional)

- A sturdy backpack loaded with heavy items such as weights, books, canned goods, or similar items to increase resistance.

Performing the single-leg heel lift

Starting position

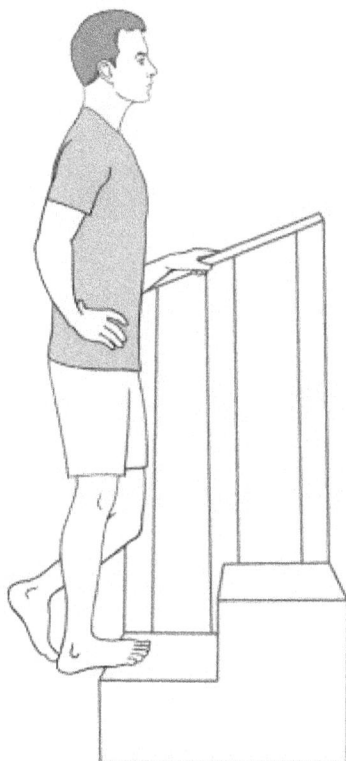

- Stand with the ball of one foot on the edge of the step and your heel off the edge. Your toes are pointed straight forward, and your knee is straight.

- The opposite leg is hanging freely off the edge of the step, and one hand is lightly placed on a wall or rail for balance.

- Lower your body by dropping the heel of the foot that's on the step while keeping your knee straight.

Movement to ending position

- With your knee straight, lift your heel up high without leaning forward. Make sure to breathe throughout the movement.

Ending position

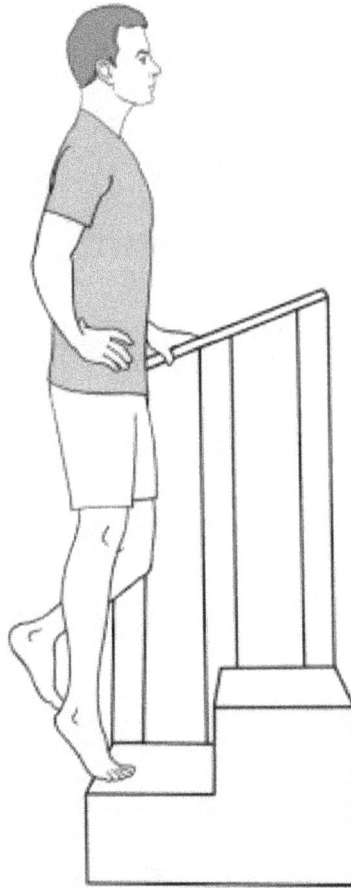

- You are on your toes with your heels lifted up high. Your toes remain pointed straight forward with your knee straight.

Return to starting position

- Lower your heel back to the starting position with control.

Repetitions

- Repeat the movement at a moderate pace on the same leg up to 15 times. Repeat this exercise on the opposite leg once you've completed your repetitions on one side.

Points to consider

- You may tend to bend the knee when lifting the heel up, preventing your calf muscle from getting the work it needs. Make sure to keep your knee straight throughout this exercise.

- You may tend to lean forward when lifting the heel up, which also prevents your calf muscle from getting the work it needs. Make sure that your body is moving straight up and down throughout this exercise.

To decrease challenge

- If you're not strong enough to lift your heel all the way up, lift it as far as you can; you'll get stronger over time.

To increase challenge

- Perform the exercise while wearing a sturdy backpack loaded with heavy items to increase the resistance.

In this chapter, you learned the nuts and bolts of performing Big Three Level III. The next chapter provides detailed instructions for Big Three Level IV.

Action Steps

- If this is the right level for you, spend some time going through the steps of each exercise until the movement feels natural. Try to cultivate an experimental mindset, and slow things down to learn the movements correctly. It's okay if your performance is less than perfect at first. Notice what "right" feels like in your body as you start to get the hang of each exercise.

- If you haven't done so already, get the exercise illustrations for this level, included in the free bonus resources at www.sixminutefitness.com/bonus. Post the illustrations on the wall in the room where you'll be exercising so you can see them easily.

21. Big Three Level IV

Level IV consists of upper body exercises designed for older adults after they have completed eight weeks of Level II or Level III lower-body training.

I recommend exclusively working your lower body in the beginning because, as we discussed in part 1, healthy, strong hips and legs are what allow you to safely stand upright and to walk—in other words, to be self-sufficient. While having a weak upper body can be inconvenient, a weak lower body negatively impacts your overall quality of life more.

After eight weeks of exclusively working your lower body, start working your upper body once daily using the exercises in this chapter. In other words, continue exercising your lower body and add the upper body exercises to your routine. Ideally, you would work your upper body immediately after you work your lower body.

This is the only level at which you will exercise only once daily.

Exercise 1: One-Arm Bent Row

The first exercise in Level IV is the one-arm bent row. This exercise primarily works the large muscles of your upper and middle back and the biceps muscle at the front of your upper arm.

Poor posture is often due to weakness in our back muscles. This weakness can cause a rounding of our upper spine, resulting in the classic "hunched over" appearance. The one-arm row helps to strengthen and stabilize nearly all the muscles involved in maintaining an upright posture without causing much strain on your lower back.

Equipment

Required

- A sturdy table or countertop.

- A weight, such as a dumbbell or ankle weight; sturdy backpack loaded with heavy items; or anything with resistance that you can hold in your hand.

To decrease challenge (optional)

- A lighter resistance.

To increase challenge (optional)

- A heavier resistance.

Performing the one-arm bent row

Starting position

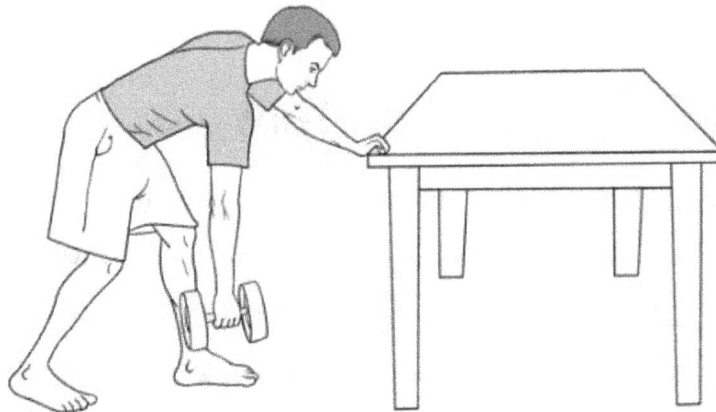

- Stand in front of a sturdy table or countertop, bending about 45 degrees forward at your waist with your back straight. One hand should be supporting you on the table or counter, and the elbow of that supporting arm should be straight. With your other hand, hold the weight or backpack hanging naturally down toward the ground.

- Your feet should be in a staggered stance, with the foot on the same side as the supporting arm forward, and the foot on the same side as the arm holding the weight or backpack one to two feet backward.

- Keep your body stable by tightening your abdominal muscles.

Movement to ending position

- Pull the weight or backpack up to the side of your body below your chest. Make sure to breathe throughout the movement.

Ending position

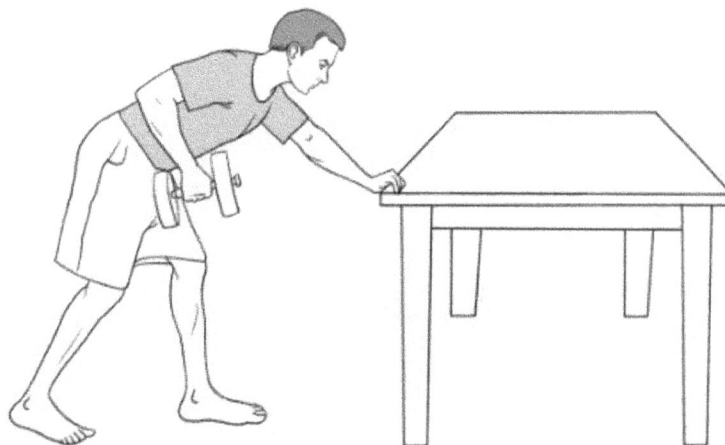

- Your body should remain stable with your abdominal muscles tight and the arm holding the weight or backpack at the side of your body below your chest. Hold for a half second.

Return to starting position

- Lower your arm back to the starting position with control.

Repetitions

- Repeat the movement at a moderate pace on the same arm up to 15 times. Repeat this exercise on the opposite arm once you've completed your repetitions on one side.

Points to consider

- Make sure your back is straight while performing this exercise. The tendency is to round the back instead of bending at the waist.

- You can place more of your body weight on the arm that is supporting you on the table or countertop if you have low back problems.

To decrease challenge

- Use a lighter resistance.

To increase challenge

- Use a heavier resistance.

Exercise 2: Floor Press

The second exercise in Level IV is the floor press. This exercise primarily works the large muscles of your chest and your triceps muscle at the back of your upper arm without causing much strain on your shoulders.

The floor press helps with daily activities, such as pushing shopping carts and heavy doors. If you happen to take a fall, you'll have an easier time pushing yourself off the ground. This exercise is also beneficial for sports such as swimming, tennis, and golf.

You'll be performing the floor press while lying on your back. I recommend performing this exercise on a firm surface, but a softer bed or couch will work if that is not available. Lying on the floor is okay if you don't have any issues getting back up.

Equipment

Required

- A pair of weights, such as dumbbells, ankle weights, or jugs of water (with handles); sturdy backpacks loaded with heavy items; or anything with resistance that you can hold in your hands.

To decrease challenge (optional)

- A lighter resistance.

To increase challenge (optional)

- A heavier resistance.

Performing the floor press

Starting position

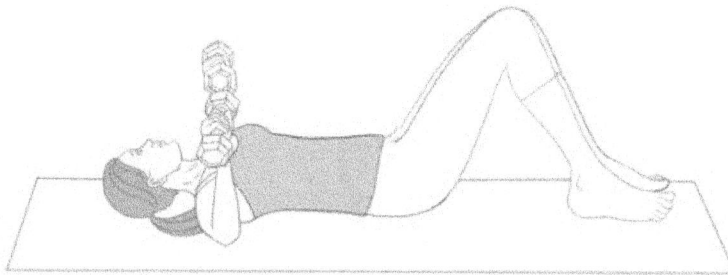

- Lie flat on your back with your knees bent and the soles of your feet flat on the surface while holding a weight in each hand.

- Your elbows should be bent at 90 degrees and resting on the surface with the weights above your chest.

- Keep your body stable by tightening your abdominal muscles.

Movement to ending position

- Push the weights up until your arms are straight but not locked out. Make sure to breathe throughout the movement.

Ending position

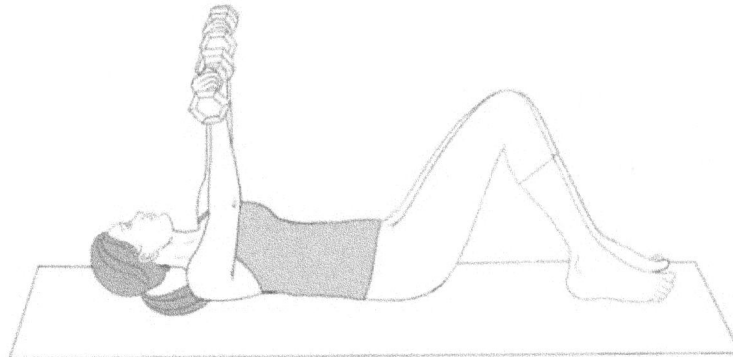

- Your body should remain stable with your abdominal muscles tight, the weights above your chest, and the arms straight but not locked out. Hold for a half second.

Return to starting position

- Lower your arms back to the starting position with control.

Repetitions

- Repeat the movement at a moderate pace up to 15 times.

Points to consider

- Make sure that your elbows are straight but not locked in the ending position. Locking the elbow will take the work off the muscles.

- Also, make sure you don't arch backward with your trunk during this exercise. You might need to lower the resistance if you're having a difficult time avoiding this.

To decrease challenge

- Use a lighter resistance.

To increase challenge

- Use a heavier resistance.

Exercise 3: Shoulder Y-Raise

The third exercise in Level IV is the shoulder Y-raise. This exercise primarily works the muscles in your shoulders, which are important for any activity that involves raising your upper arms. It also works the deep rotator cuff muscles that stabilize and protect your shoulders from injury.

This exercise improves the ability to perform daily activities, such as reaching overhead to grab something from a high cupboard or lifting heavy grandchildren, with greater ease.

Equipment

Required

- A pair of weights, such as dumbbells, ankle weights, jugs of water (with handles); sturdy backpacks loaded with heavy items; or anything else with resistance that you can hold in your hands.

To decrease challenge

- A lighter resistance.

To increase challenge

- A heavier resistance.

Performing the shoulder Y-raise

Starting position

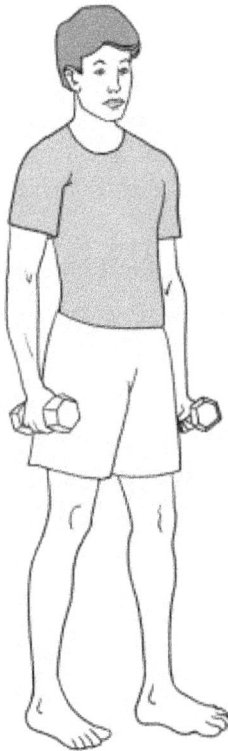

- Stand with your feet shoulder-width apart with the pair of weights in your hands, arms hanging by your side, and palms facing inwards toward your body.

- Keep your body stable by tightening your abdominal muscles.

Movement to ending position

- Lift the weights to shoulder height with your thumbs up, elbows straight, and arms at about a 30-degree angle in front of your body such that your arms form a Y shape in front of your chest. Make sure to breathe throughout the movement.

Ending position

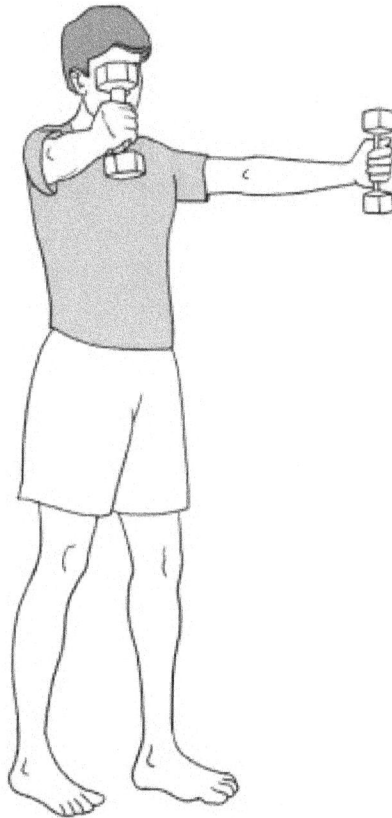

- Your body should remain stable with your abdominal muscles tight. Your arms are at shoulder height with your thumbs up, elbows straight, and arms at about a 30-degree angle in front of your body, forming a Y shape in front of your chest. Hold for a half second.

Return to starting position

- Lower your arms to the starting position with control.

Repetitions

- Repeat the movement at a moderate pace up to 15 times.

Points to consider

- Make sure you raise the arms at about a 30-degree angle in front of your body. An easy way to understand this is by holding your arms straight out to the sides and then moving them slightly together in front of your body, like you're giving a hug to a giant tree. This position is optimal for exercising your rotator cuff muscles.

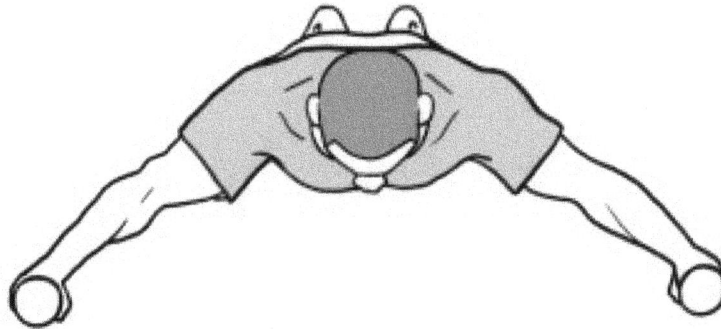

- Make sure you lift with your thumbs up. The thumb-up position creates more space inside the shoulder joint during this movement, which reduces the likelihood of causing painful jamming.

- Make sure to lift your arms no higher than the level of your shoulders. When you raise your arms higher than this, other muscles you don't want to use get involved.

- Also, make sure you don't hike up your shoulders or arch backward with your trunk during this exercise. You might need to lower the resistance if you're having a difficult time avoiding this.

To decrease challenge

- Use a lighter resistance.

To increase challenge

- Use a heavier resistance.

In this chapter, you learned the nuts and bolts of performing Big Three Level IV, and that concludes part 4. In part 5, you'll put together everything you've learned to execute the six-minute workout.

Action Steps

- Spend some time going through the steps of each exercise until the movement feels natural. Take an experimental mindset, and slow things down to learn the movements correctly. It's okay if your performance is not perfect at first. Notice what "right" feels like in your body as you start to get the hang of each exercise.

- If you haven't already done so, get the exercise illustrations for this level, included in the free bonus resources at www.sixminutefitness.com/bonus. Post the illustrations on the wall in the room where you'll be exercising so you can easily see them.

Part 5
Executing the Six-Minute Workout

This part of the book puts everything together so you can execute the six-minute workout. To do that, I provide you with eight-week workout plans for all levels of the Big Three and additional information about how to get the most from your workout.

Part 5 Topics:

- Eight-week workout plans for all levels.

- Tracking progress and overcoming plateaus.

- Adapting exercise to your ability.

- Tips for family members and caregivers helping older adults with exercise.

22. Eight-Week Workout Plans for All Levels

I promise that if you follow the program exactly as described in this book, you will see dramatic improvements in your strength, balance, and energy in 15 days. If you haven't already done so, you can get the eight-week workout plans for all levels as part of the free bonus resources at www.sixminutefitness.com/bonus (they're available in PDF, Excel, and Google Sheets formats).

Here's a review of programming considerations for the Big Three:

- **Number of exercises:** Three.

- **Sessions a day exercise is performed:** Two times a day.

- **Time spaced between sessions:** At least three hours apart; exercises should preferably be performed before meals.

- **Days a week exercise is performed:** Exercise seven days a week for the first two weeks, with exercise reduced to six days a week after that.

- **Repetitions:** Each exercise is performed for up to 15 repetitions in sequence without rest. Whatever amount of repetitions you do should be the same for all exercises within a workout session. One round is counted every time you complete all three of the exercises. Your goal is to complete as many rounds as possible in six minutes or until exhaustion.

- **Rest break:** Short rest breaks of up to 30 seconds are allowed, but only if you're completely exhausted and only after a full round of exercise has been completed.

- **Order of exercises:** This changes daily in a rotational manner. For example, on day one, you'll perform exercises in the order ABC, on day two CAB, and day three BCA.

- **Same or different routines:** Same set of exercises daily until you're ready for a higher level. If you're on the border between levels, you can perform the harder level for your first session and the easier one for your second session.

- **Upper body exercises:** Performed once daily after eight weeks of Level II or Level III.

Big Three Level I: Eight-Week Workout Plan

Level I is designed for older adults who can't stand or who have difficulty standing for at least six minutes with or without support, such as a walker, due to limitations in strength, balance, or energy.

Level I: Eight-Week Workout Plan							
	Day 1	Day 2	Day 3	Day 4	Day 5	Day 6	Day 7
WEEK 1 Session 1 & 2	Straight Leg Raise Single-Leg Tuck Hip Raise	Single-Leg Tuck Hip Raise Straight Leg Raise	Hip Raise Straight Leg Raise Singe-Leg Tuck	Straight Leg Raise Single-Leg Tuck Hip Raise	Single-Leg Tuck Hip Raise Straight Leg Raise	Hip Raise Straight Leg Raise Singe-Leg Tuck	Straight Leg Raise Single-Leg Tuck Hip Raise
WEEK 2 Session 1 & 2	Single-Leg Tuck Hip Raise Straight Leg Raise	Hip Raise Straight Leg Raise Singe-Leg Tuck	Straight Leg Raise Single-Leg Tuck Hip Raise	Single-Leg Tuck Hip Raise Straight Leg Raise	Hip Raise Straight Leg Raise Singe-Leg Tuck	Straight Leg Raise Single-Leg Tuck Hip Raise	Single-Leg Tuck Hip Raise Straight Leg Raise
WEEK 3 & 6 Session 1 & 2	Hip Raise Straight Leg Raise Singe-Leg Tuck	Straight Leg Raise Single-Leg Tuck Hip Raise	Single-Leg Tuck Hip Raise Straight Leg Raise	Hip Raise Straight Leg Raise Singe-Leg Tuck	Straight Leg Raise Single-Leg Tuck Hip Raise	Single-Leg Tuck Hip Raise Straight Leg Raise	Rest Day
WEEK 4 & 7 Session 1 & 2	Straight Leg Raise Single-Leg Tuck Hip Raise	Single-Leg Tuck Hip Raise Straight Leg Raise	Hip Raise Straight Leg Raise Singe-Leg Tuck	Straight Leg Raise Single-Leg Tuck Hip Raise	Single-Leg Tuck Hip Raise Straight Leg Raise	Hip Raise Straight Leg Raise Singe-Leg Tuck	Rest Day
WEEK 5 & 8 Session 1 & 2	Single-Leg Tuck Hip Raise Straight Leg Raise	Hip Raise Straight Leg Raise Singe-Leg Tuck	Straight Leg Raise Single-Leg Tuck Hip Raise	Single-Leg Tuck Hip Raise Straight Leg Raise	Hip Raise Straight Leg Raise Singe-Leg Tuck	Straight Leg Raise Single-Leg Tuck Hip Raise	Rest Day

Note: After 8 weeks you can move to Level II or repeat weeks 6-8.

Big Three Level II: Eight-Week Workout Plan

Level II is designed for older adults who have no difficulty standing but who lack the strength or energy to walk at a vigorous pace for at least six minutes.

This level is also designed for those who have difficulty going up and down a flight of stairs.

	Level II: Eight-Week Workout Plan						
	Day 1	Day 2	Day 3	Day 4	Day 5	Day 6	Day 7
WEEK 1 Session 1 & 2	Chair Squat Heel Lift High Knees Marching	Heel Lift High Knees Marching Chair Squat	High Knees Marching Chair Squat Heel Lift	Chair Squat Heel Lift High Knees Marching	Heel Lift High Knees Marching Chair Squat	High Knees Marching Chair Squat Heel Lift	Chair Squat Heel Lift High Knees Marching
WEEK 2 Session 1 & 2	Heel Lift High Knees Marching Chair Squat	High Knees Marching Chair Squat Heel Lift	Chair Squat Heel Lift High Knees Marching	Heel Lift High Knees Marching Chair Squat	High Knees Marching Chair Squat Heel Lift	Chair Squat Heel Lift High Knees Marching	Heel Lift High Knees Marching Chair Squat
WEEK 3 & 6 Session 1 & 2	High Knees Marching Chair Squat Heel Lift	Chair Squat Heel Lift High Knees Marching	Heel Lift High Knees Marching Chair Squat	High Knees Marching Chair Squat Heel Lift	Chair Squat Heel Lift High Knees Marching	Heel Lift High Knees Marching Chair Squat	Rest Day
WEEK 4 & 7 Session 1 & 2	Chair Squat Heel Lift High Knees Marching	Heel Lift High Knees Marching Chair Squat	High Knees Marching Chair Squat Heel Lift	Chair Squat Heel Lift High Knees Marching	Heel Lift High Knees Marching Chair Squat	High Knees Marching Chair Squat Heel Lift	Rest Day
WEEK 5 & 8 Session 1 & 2	Heel Lift High Knees Marching Chair Squat	High Knees Marching Chair Squat Heel Lift	Chair Squat Heel Lift High Knees Marching	Heel Lift High Knees Marching Chair Squat	High Knees Marching Chair Squat Heel Lift	Chair Squat Heel Lift High Knees Marching	Rest Day

Note: After 8 weeks you can move to Level III or repeat weeks 6-8.

Big Three Level III: Eight-Week Workout Plan

Level III is designed for older adults who are high functioning. This means they can walk at a vigorous pace for more than six minutes and can go up and down several flights of stairs with no difficulty.

Level III: Eight-Week Workout Plan

	Day 1	Day 2	Day 3	Day 4	Day 5	Day 6	Day 7
WEEK 1 Session 1 & 2	Stationary Lunge Step-Up Single-Leg Heel Lift	Step-Up Single-Leg Heel Lift Stationary Lunge	Single-Leg Heel Lift Stationary Lunge Step-Up	Stationary Lunge Step-Up Single-Leg Heel Lift	Step-Up Single-Leg Heel Lift Stationary Lunge	Single-Leg Heel Lift Stationary Lunge Step-Up	Stationary Lunge Step-Up Single-Leg Heel Lift
WEEK 2 Session 1 & 2	Step-Up Single-Leg Heel Lift Stationary Lunge	Single-Leg Heel Lift Stationary Lunge Step-Up	Stationary Lunge Step-Up Single-Leg Heel Lift	Step-Up Single-Leg Heel Lift Stationary Lunge	Single-Leg Heel Lift Stationary Lunge Step-Up	Stationary Lunge Step-Up Single-Leg Heel Lift	Step-Up Single-Leg Heel Lift Stationary Lunge
WEEK 3 & 6 Session 1 & 2	Single-Leg Heel Lift Stationary Lunge Step-Up	Stationary Lunge Step-Up Single-Leg Heel Lift	Step-Up Single-Leg Heel Lift Stationary Lunge	Single-Leg Heel Lift Stationary Lunge Step-Up	Stationary Lunge Step-Up Single-Leg Heel Lift	Step-Up Single-Leg Heel Lift Stationary Lunge	Rest Day
WEEK 4 & 7 Session 1 & 2	Stationary Lunge Step-Up Single-Leg Heel Lift	Step-Up Single-Leg Heel Lift Stationary Lunge	Single-Leg Heel Lift Stationary Lunge Step-Up	Stationary Lunge Step-Up Single-Leg Heel Lift	Step-Up Single-Leg Heel Lift Stationary Lunge	Single-Leg Heel Lift Stationary Lunge Step-Up	Rest Day
WEEK 5 & 8 Session 1 & 2	Step-Up Single-Leg Heel Lift Stationary Lunge	Single-Leg Heel Lift Stationary Lunge Step-Up	Stationary Lunge Step-Up Single-Leg Heel Lift	Step-Up Single-Leg Heel Lift Stationary Lunge	Single-Leg Heel Lift Stationary Lunge Step-Up	Stationary Lunge Step-Up Single-Leg Heel Lift	Rest Day

Note: After 8 weeks you can repeat weeks 6-8.

Big Three Level IV: Eight-Week Workout Plan

Level IV consists of upper body exercises designed for older adults after they have completed eight weeks of Level II or Level III training.

Level VI: Eight-Week Workout Plan

	Day 1	Day 2	Day 3	Day 4	Day 5	Day 6	Day 7
WEEK 1 Session 1	One-Arm Bent Row Floor Press Shoulder Y-Raise	Floor Press Shoulder Y-Raise One-Arm Bent Row	Shoulder Y-Raise One-Arm Bent Row Floor Press	One-Arm Bent Row Floor Press Shoulder Y-Raise	Floor Press Shoulder Y-Raise One-Arm Bent Row	Shoulder Y-Raise One-Arm Bent Row Floor Press	One-Arm Bent Row Floor Press Shoulder Y-Raise
WEEK 2 Session 1	Floor Press Shoulder Y-Raise One-Arm Bent Row	Shoulder Y-Raise One-Arm Bent Row Floor Press	One-Arm Bent Row Floor Press Shoulder Y-Raise	Floor Press Shoulder Y-Raise One-Arm Bent Row	Shoulder Y-Raise One-Arm Bent Row Floor Press	One-Arm Bent Row Floor Press Shoulder Y-Raise	Floor Press Shoulder Y-Raise One-Arm Bent Row
WEEK 3 & 6 Session 1	Shoulder Y-Raise One-Arm Bent Row Floor Press	One-Arm Bent Row Floor Press Shoulder Y-Raise	Floor Press Shoulder Y-Raise One-Arm Bent Row	Shoulder Y-Raise One-Arm Bent Row Floor Press	One-Arm Bent Row Floor Press Shoulder Y-Raise	Floor Press Shoulder Y-Raise One-Arm Bent Row	Rest Day
WEEK 4 & 7 Session 1	One-Arm Bent Row Floor Press Shoulder Y-Raise	Floor Press Shoulder Y-Raise One-Arm Bent Row	Shoulder Y-Raise One-Arm Bent Row Floor Press	One-Arm Bent Row Floor Press Shoulder Y-Raise	Floor Press Shoulder Y-Raise One-Arm Bent Row	Shoulder Y-Raise One-Arm Bent Row Floor Press	Rest Day
WEEK 5 & 8 Session 1	Floor Press Shoulder Y-Raise One-Arm Bent Row	Shoulder Y-Raise One-Arm Bent Row Floor Press	One-Arm Bent Row Floor Press Shoulder Y-Raise	Floor Press Shoulder Y-Raise One-Arm Bent Row	Shoulder Y-Raise One-Arm Bent Row Floor Press	One-Arm Bent Row Floor Press Shoulder Y-Raise	Rest Day

Note: After 8 weeks you can repeat weeks 6-8.

Action Steps

- Make sure you've downloaded the eight-week workout plans included in the free bonus resources: www.sixminutefitness.com/bonus. Post the workout plan for your level on the wall in the room where you'll be exercising so you can see it easily.

23. Track Your Progress and Break Through Plateaus

Tracking your progress is one of the most important ways to figure out when something's working and when it isn't. It's also how you'll know when you've hit a workout plateau.

A plateau is when you stall out on progress despite continuing to do "all of the right things." Your body has either adapted to the exercise you've been performing for a while and needs a different workout, or your body is fatigued from overtraining and needs additional rest in order to progress.

By tracking your progress, you'll know if any of these issues are plaguing your workout, and I'll show you how to troubleshoot them to ensure that you keep going on the right path.

Tracking Progress

Bonnie Blair—one of the top skaters of her era and one of the most decorated athletes in Olympic history—once said, "Winning does not always mean being first. Winning means you are doing better than you have done before."[51] Similarly, with exercise, success is not measured by whether you reach or surpass your fitness goals on a particular day. Rather, it's measured by the small, incremental changes you experience during exercise that let you know you're doing better than you did before.

The best way to see these changes is by tracking your workout progress. When you track your progress, you know what was accomplished in a workout, and then you can figure out when something's working and when it isn't. Tracking your progress also helps keep you motivated and accountable with exercise and makes it more likely that you will reach and even surpass your fitness goals.

It's simple to track progress. I recommend keeping track of the three Rs: repetitions, rounds, and rest.

Repetitions

Keep track of the number of repetitions you performed during your workouts. While each Big Three exercise is performed for up to 15 repetitions in sequence without rest, you may not be ready for that at the start. Whatever amount of repetitions you do should be the same for all exercises within a workout session.

For example, if you decide to do eight repetitions of each exercise, keep track of this number and note when you feel ready to increase it, then track your progress against the new number. Then repeat. Your goal is to gradually work your way up to 15 repetitions.

Rounds

Keep track of the number of rounds you performed during your workouts. One round is counted every time you complete each of the three exercises in the Big Three.

Keep track of how many rounds you complete during your six-minute workout session. Your goal is to perform progressively more rounds over time.

Rest

Keep track of how many rounds you've completed before needing to rest during your workouts. Short rest breaks of up to 30 seconds are allowed at the end of a full round of exercise.

Keep track of how many rounds you complete in each session before taking your first rest break. Your goal is to perform progressively more rounds over time without rest and eventually eliminate rest altogether.

By tracking your progress, you'll notice the three Rs improve rapidly during the first two weeks of exercise if you're following the seven strategies for unlocking your fitness potential that I described in part 2. For most people, the rate of improvement tends to slow down a little after the first two weeks, but you should continue to see changes until week eight and beyond.

If you notice the three Rs stall for two weeks or more, you might have hit a workout plateau. Let's now look at how to break through those plateaus.

Breaking Through Plateaus

So, what do you do when you see no progress? It depends on where you are in your workout. We'll explore what to do when you see no progress at three different stages: after the first two weeks, between week two and week eight, and after week eight.

First two weeks

You should see the three Rs improve rapidly during the first two weeks of exercise. But what if you don't notice any improvements during this stage of the program? It's unlikely that you've hit a plateau at this point because you're so early in the program, and plateaus typically happen after you've been exercising for several weeks or more. Likely, you need to revisit the fundamentals of exercise to make sure they're in line.

First, review the seven strategies for unlocking your fitness potential in part 2, and make sure you're following each of them.

Second, review chapter 17 and make sure you're also following the suggestions for personalization, precision, and programming.

If this doesn't resolve the issue, see if changing the level of the workout will help. Doing these things will resolve most cases of lack of progress during the first two weeks.

Between week two and week eight

What if you notice no improvements for two consecutive weeks between week two and week eight of the program? It's normal for improvements to slow down a little after the first two weeks, but you should continue to see changes until week eight and beyond.

If you're not making progress and you're feeling more fatigued than usual, you might be overtraining. This is a common reason for a plateau, and the most effective thing to do to overcome this is to rest. Take an entire week off from performing the exercises before picking up where you left off. After resting for a week, you should immediately start to see improvements.

If you're feeling good, go through the same steps as in the first two weeks. Also make sure nothing has changed in your life that may impact your progress, such as:

- **Sleep:** Exercise performance will be impacted negatively if you're not sleeping enough or not sleeping well.

- **Physical activity outside of exercise:** You may be more tired during exercise if you have more going on throughout your day.

- **Changes to medications or health:** Changes in your medications and health condition may negatively impact exercise performance.

If factors outside of exercise are impacting your workout progress, keep exercising unless your doctor tells you otherwise. Doing something is better than doing nothing, and you'll be better off if or when these factors are no longer an issue.

After week eight

What if you notice no improvements for two consecutive weeks after week eight of the program? Again, it's normal for improvements to slow down a bit after the first two weeks, but you should continue to see changes even beyond eight weeks.

Go through the same steps as you did between week two and week eight. If none of the problems listed apply, or if none of the solutions fix the problem, it might be a sign that your body needs something different for it to continue changing; plateaus can also happen when your body has adjusted to the demands of your workout and are a sign that you need something different to continue progressing.

If you're on Level I or II, try replacing one session a day with a higher level, or move on entirely to a higher level. If you're on Level II or Level III, you can replace one session a day with a lower level to give your body something different to improve your progress.

On the other hand, a workout plateau after eight weeks might not be a big deal if you're happy with your progress and don't feel that you need additional strength, energy, and balance. If this is the case, you can maintain your current level of function without losing any of the gains you've made by exercising one session a day for four or five days a week.

Now that you can identify and troubleshoot issues that may plague your progress, you can sail through the program unless you have some physical limitations. In the next chapter, I'll show you how to adapt exercise to any physical limitations you may have.

Action Step

- Track the three Rs in a notebook. You'll find a place on the bottom right side of the printable eight-week workout plan where you can track the three Rs. Notice the progress you're making, and also notice if you've made no progress for two consecutive weeks. If so, use the information in this chapter to help keep you going on the right path.

24. Adapting Exercise to Physical Limitations

You may have limitations that prevent you from performing an exercise with the technique I've instructed or even from performing an exercise at all. But don't worry. It's okay to adapt the exercises in this book to what works for you and to disregard an exercise entirely if needed. Doing something is better than doing nothing.

For example, if you're unable to point your feet straight forward on a standing exercise, like the heel lift, because of a physical limitation, don't worry about it. If it's been cleared by your doctor, perform the exercise in whatever manner works for you.

If you have had a stroke and are paralyzed on an entire side of your body, perform the exercise only on the side you do have control over. If you can perform an exercise only with assistance due to a lack of strength or some other reason, you can ask a family member or caregiver to help. However, the assistance provided should be the minimum needed for you to perform the exercise so your body can get as much work as possible.

Exercising regularly is one of the best things you can do for your body and your health. Soon after you start this program, you'll begin to see and feel the benefits that physical activity can have on your well-being.

I want this program to work for you, and doing something is better than doing nothing, so feel free to adapt the exercises to whatever works for you and modify the program to accommodate your limitations.

But it isn't just physical limitations that may stand in your way, so in the next chapter I'll provide tips for family members and caregivers helping older adults with memory issues or who lack the motivation to exercise.

Action Steps

- Look at the exercises you would like to perform, and see if you need to adapt or eliminate any from your workout.

- Are there any exercises you can perform but only with assistance due to a lack of strength or some other reason? If so, ask for help from a family member or caregiver.

25. Tips for Family Members and Caregivers

Older adults with memory issues or who lack the motivation to exercise will need help from another person.

Although we never want to force someone to exercise when they don't want to, persuasion is sometimes necessary because a persistent lack of movement leads to serious issues, such as debility, bed sores, and injuries from falls.

Older adults with memory issues or who lack motivation may have a difficult time starting and sticking with an exercise program. But I've found it becomes less challenging once exercise becomes routine, and changes in strength, balance, and energy become apparent after a few weeks.

The key to persuasion is a simple process I've created called the four Es: enthusiasm, empathy, encouragement, and ease. This process takes only a few minutes and has been effective with even my most exercise-resistant clients. Let's explore each step in detail.

Enthusiasm

Richard Simmons, the semi-retired American fitness instructor known for his eccentric and energetic personality, is a great example of enthusiasm at its best. It's difficult not to feel pumped up and motivated to move when you watch him.

So the first step in motivating someone is to be enthusiastic. Your enthusiasm is contagious, and it can shift another person's energy level and desire to exercise in powerful ways. To make enthusiasm work, you have to authentically feel it and express it in your words and body language.

Try to authentically feel and express enthusiasm in your voice, posture, gesture, and facial expression while saying something like, "Dad, it's time to exercise. It'll only take six minutes, and you'll feel great afterward. Let's do it!" If you encounter any resistance, move to the next step.

Empathy

The second step is to feel and express empathy: the ability to understand and share the feelings of another. It's important because a person is more likely to be open to your suggestions when they know you've understood and considered their perspective.

So to feel empathetic, you should know the common reasons why an older adult may not want to exercise: They may have lost hope that things will ever get better. They may be fearful that the aches and pains they experience daily will get worse if they exercise. They may feel constantly exhausted and don't know if they have the energy needed to exercise.

Whatever the reason, start by stepping into their shoes and feel what they may be feeling. Then express your understanding through your words and body language. Try to authentically feel and express empathy in your voice, posture, gesture, and facial expression while saying something like, "Dad, I can understand that you're feeling exhausted, and the aches that come with your age don't help. I also wonder if you've lost some hope that things can get better." It helps to pause for several seconds at this point to tune in to feelings that may be coming up for you and the other person. Then, move to the next step, which is to encourage the person.

Encourage

After feeling and expressing empathy, it's time to encourage the person to exercise.

For this to be effective, I suggest doing two things. First, understand the person's personal values and bring them into this step. A person's values can be things like determination or hope or respecting authority figures such as doctors. Second, remind the person of the benefits of exercise that are important to them. These benefits can be things like feeling more energized after exercising, gaining the ability to live more independently, feeling happier because they can avoid hospitalizations, or having more energy playing with the grandchildren.

Whatever the reason for exercising, keep it positive, and express it with passion in your words and body language.

Use this step to authentically feel and express passion in your voice, posture, gesture, and facial expression while saying something like, "Dad, you always told us growing up that sometimes things will get worse before they get better, and having hope will get you through these times. It's no different getting your body working better through exercise. Remember how much you want to get back to gardening? What do you say?" If the person still isn't convinced to exercise at this point, it's time for the final step.

Ease

The fourth and final step is to ease into exercise. Use this when the previous steps haven't persuaded the person to take action. Your goal is to make exercise something the person can try for a few repetitions to see how it feels, knowing they can stop any time.

To make this step work, I recommend you first openly acknowledge that the person really doesn't want to exercise. Then suggest that they try just a few repetitions of one exercise to see how it feels. Tell them they can stop any time.

Perform this step with enthusiasm, and encourage the person to continue exercising after they've started. With enthusiastic encouragement, most people won't stop exercising once they've begun and may even surprise you with their new motivation.

Use this step to authentically feel and express enthusiasm in your voice, posture, gesture, and facial expression while saying something like, "I totally understand that the idea of exercise doesn't sit well with you right now, but let's just do five chair squats and see how it feels. I'll help you, and you can stop any time if you don't want to continue after that. Come on, let's start now."

As the person approaches the fifth repetition of the exercise, enthusiastically encourage them to continue by saying something like, "Wow, you're looking really strong! I'm amazed by how well you're doing! Keep going, I know you've got it in you!"

Applying the four Es takes only a few minutes and has been effective with even my most exercise-resistant clients. However, at times, nothing you do will persuade someone to exercise. It's best to yield to the person's wishes in these moments.

Fortunately, just two or three good workout sessions a week is enough to see improvements with this program in most adults. That may be all you will get out of someone who really doesn't like to exercise—but after a few weeks, they may be more motivated after noticing improvements in their strength, balance, and energy. So stay positive and be patient!

Action Steps

- If you're a family member or a caregiver for an older adult you'd like to help with exercise, practice the four Es a few times on your own to get comfortable with the method before using it to persuade them to exercise

Conclusion

Congratulations on completing 6-Minute Fitness at 60+!

I hope you'll use what you've learned in this book to move, feel, and live better than you ever have before.

Remember, consistency is the key to your fitness goals. Stay motivated and stay consistent! If you do, I promise you will achieve the strength, balance, and energy you've envisioned.

References

[←1]

Wade, Alison. "Watch: 95-Year-Old Man Sets 200 Meter Age Group World Record." Runner's World. March 10, 2015. Accessed August 25, 2020. https://www.runnersworld.com/advanced/a20851308/watch-95-year-old-man-sets-200-meter-age-group-world-record/.

[←2]

Peterson, Mark D., Ananda Sen, and Paul M. Gordon. "Influence of Resistance Exercise on Lean Body Mass in Aging Adults: A Meta-Analysis." Medicine and Science in Sports and Exercise 43, no. 2 (February 2011): 249–58.

[←3]

Csapo, R., and L. M. Alegre. "Effects of Resistance Training with Moderate vs Heavy Loads on Muscle Mass and Strength in the Elderly: A Meta-Analysis." Scandinavian Journal of Medicine & Science in Sports 26, no. 9 (September 2016): 995–1006..

[←4]

Bickel, C. Scott, James M. Cross, and Marcas M. Bamman. "Exercise Dosing to Retain Resistance Training Adaptations in Young and Older Adults." Medicine and Science in Sports and Exercise 43, no. 7 (July 2011): 1177–87.

[←5]

Starkweather, Angela R., Areej A. Alhaeeri, Alison Montpetit, Jenni Brumelle, Kristin Filler, Marty Montpetit, Lathika Mohanraj, Debra E. Lyon, and Colleen K. Jackson-Cook. "An Integrative Review of Factors Associated with Telomere Length and Implications for Biobehavioral Research." Nursing Research 63, no. 1 (2014): 36–50.

[←6]

Cherkas, Lynn F., Janice L. Hunkin, Bernet S. Kato, J. Brent Richards, Jeffrey P. Gardner, Gabriela L. Surdulescu, Masayuki Kimura, Xiaobin Lu, Tim D. Spector, and Abraham Aviv. "The Association between Physical Activity in Leisure Time and Leukocyte Telomere Length." Archives of Internal Medicine 168, no. 2 (January 28, 2008): 154–58.

[←7]

Ibid.

[←8]

Robinson, Matthew M., Surendra Dasari, Adam R. Konopka, Matthew L. Johnson, S. Manjunatha, Raul Ruiz Esponda, Rickey E. Carter, Ian R. Lanza, and K. Sreekumaran Nair. "Enhanced Protein Translation Underlies Improved Metabolic and Physical Adaptations to Different Exercise Training Modes in Young and Old Humans." Cell Metabolism 25, no. 3 (07 2017): 581–92.

[←9]

Chen, Feng-Tzu, Jennifer L. Etnier, Kuei-Hui Chan, Ping-Kun Chiu, Tsung-Ming Hung, and Yu-Kai Chang. "Effects of Exercise Training Interventions on Executive Function in Older Adults: A Systematic Review and Meta-Analysis." Sports Medicine (Auckland, N.Z.), May 23, 2020. Mora, Jorge Camilo, and Willy M. Valencia. "Exercise and Older Adults." Clinics in Geriatric Medicine 34, no. 1 (2018): 145–62. Schuch, Felipe B., Davy Vancampfort, Justin Richards, Simon Rosenbaum, Philip B. Ward, and Brendon Stubbs. "Exercise as a Treatment for Depression: A Meta-Analysis Adjusting for Publication Bias." Journal of Psychiatric Research 77 (June 2016): 42–51.

[←10]

Bouaziz, Walid, Alexandra Malgoyre, Elise Schmitt, Pierre-Olivier Lang, Thomas Vogel, and Lukshe Kanagaratnam. "Effect of High-Intensity Interval Training and Continuous Endurance Training on Peak Oxygen Uptake among Seniors Aged 65 or Older: A Meta-Analysis of Randomized Controlled Trials." International Journal of Clinical Practice 74, no. 6 (June 2020): e13490.

[←11]

Blackwell, James E. M., Brett Doleman, Philip J. J. Herrod, Samuel Ricketts, Bethan E. Phillips, Jonathan N. Lund, and John P. Williams. "Short-Term (<8 Wk) High-Intensity Interval Training in Diseased Cohorts." Medicine and Science in Sports and Exercise 50, no. 9 (2018): 1740–49. Liu, Jing-Xin, Lin Zhu, Pei-Jun Li, Ning Li, and Yan-Bing Xu. "Effectiveness of High-Intensity Interval Training on Glycemic Control and Cardiorespiratory Fitness in Patients with Type 2 Diabetes: A Systematic Review and Meta-Analysis." Aging Clinical and Experimental Research 31, no. 5 (May 2019): 575–93. Wiener, Joshua, Amanda McIntyre, Scott Janssen, Jeffrey Ty Chow, Cristina Batey, and Robert Teasell. "Effectiveness of High-Intensity Interval Training for Fitness and Mobility Post Stroke: A Systematic Review." PM & R: The Journal of Injury, Function, and Rehabilitation 11, no. 8 (2019): 868–78. Wisløff, Ulrik, Asbjørn Støylen, Jan P. Loennechen, Morten Bruvold, Øivind Rognmo, Per Magnus Haram, Arnt Erik Tjønna, et al. "Superior Cardiovascular Effect of Aerobic Interval Training versus Moderate Continuous Training in Heart Failure Patients: A Randomized Study." Circulation 115, no. 24 (June 19, 2007): 3086–94.

[←12]

Grace, Fergal, Peter Herbert, Adrian D. Elliott, Jo Richards, Alexander Beaumont, and Nicholas F. Sculthorpe. "High Intensity Interval Training (HIIT) Improves Resting Blood Pressure, Metabolic (MET) Capacity and Heart Rate Reserve without Compromising Cardiac Function in Sedentary Aging Men." Experimental Gerontology 109 (2018): 75–81.

[←13]

Burgomaster, Kirsten A., Scott C. Hughes, George J. F. Heigenhauser, Suzanne N. Bradwell, and Martin J. Gibala. "Six Sessions of Sprint Interval Training Increases Muscle Oxidative Potential and Cycle Endurance Capacity in Humans." Journal of Applied Physiology (Bethesda, Md.: 1985) 98, no. 6 (June 2005): 1985–90.

[←14]

Cortell-Tormo, Juan M., Pablo Tercedor Sánchez, Ivan Chulvi-Medrano, Juan Tortosa-Martínez, Carmen Manchado-López, Salvador Llana-Belloch, and Pedro Pérez-Soriano. "Effects of Functional Resistance Training on Fitness and Quality of Life in Females with Chronic Nonspecific Low-Back Pain." Journal of Back and Musculoskeletal Rehabilitation 31, no. 1 (February 6, 2018): 95–105. Haddock, Christopher K., Walker S. C. Poston, Katie M. Heinrich, Sara A. Jahnke, and Nattinee Jitnarin. "The Benefits of High-Intensity Functional Training Fitness Programs for Military Personnel." Military Medicine 181, no. 11 (2016): e1508–14. Peterson, James A. "10 Nice-to-Know Facts About Functional Training." ACSM's Health & Fitness Journal 17, no. 5 (October 2013): 48.

[←15]

Toots, Annika, Håkan Littbrand, Nina Lindelöf, Robert Wiklund, Henrik Holmberg, Peter Nordström, Lillemor Lundin-Olsson, Yngve Gustafson, and Erik Rosendahl. "Effects of a High-Intensity Functional Exercise Program on Dependence in Activities of Daily Living and Balance in Older Adults with Dementia." Journal of the American Geriatrics Society 64, no. 1 (January 2016): 55–64.

[←16]

Thompson, Christian J., Karen Myers Cobb, and John Blackwell. "Functional Training Improves Club Head Speed and Functional Fitness in Older Golfers." Journal of Strength and Conditioning Research 21, no. 1 (February 2007): 131–37.

[←17]

Blair, S. N., H. W. Kohl, R. S. Paffenbarger, D. G. Clark, K. H. Cooper, and L. W. Gibbons. "Physical Fitness and All-Cause Mortality. A Prospective Study of Healthy Men and Women." JAMA 262, no. 17 (November 3, 1989): 2395–2401.

[←18]

Garber, Carol Ewing, Bryan Blissmer, Michael R. Deschenes, Barry A. Franklin, Michael J. Lamonte, I.-Min Lee, David C. Nieman, David P. Swain, and American College of Sports Medicine. "American College of Sports Medicine Position Stand. Quantity and Quality of Exercise for Developing and Maintaining Cardiorespiratory, Musculoskeletal, and Neuromotor Fitness in Apparently Healthy Adults: Guidance for Prescribing Exercise." Medicine and Science in Sports and Exercise 43, no. 7 (July 2011): 1334–59..

[←19]

Thompson, Walter R. ACSM's Guidelines for Exercise Testing and Prescription. Lippincott Williams & Wilkins, 2010.

[←20]

Centers for Disease Control and Prevention (CDC). "Vital Signs: Walking among Adults—United States, 2005 and 2010." MMWR. Morbidity and Mortality Weekly Report 61, no. 31 (August 10, 2012): 595–601.

[←21]

Fink, Julius, Brad Jon Schoenfeld, and Koichi Nakazato. "The Role of Hormones in Muscle Hypertrophy." The Physician and Sportsmedicine 46, no. 1 (2018): 129–34. Kraemer, William J., and Nicholas A. Ratamess. "Hormonal Responses and Adaptations to Resistance Exercise and Training." Sports Medicine (Auckland, N.Z.) 35, no. 4 (2005): 339–61.

[←22]

Sellami, Maha, Nicola Luigi Bragazzi, Maamer Slimani, Lawrence Hayes, Georges Jabbour, Andrea De Giorgio, and Benoit Dugué. "The Effect of Exercise on Glucoregulatory Hormones: A Countermeasure to Human Aging: Insights from a Comprehensive Review of the Literature." International Journal of Environmental Research and Public Health 16, no. 10 (15 2019).

[←23]

Melmed, Shlomo. Williams Textbook of Endocrinology, 2020.

[←24]

Magutah, Karani, Kihumbu Thairu, and Nilesh Patel. "Effect of Short Moderate Intensity Exercise Bouts on Cardiovascular Function and Maximal Oxygen Consumption in Sedentary Older Adults." BMJ Open Sport & Exercise Medicine 6, no. 1 (2020): e000672. Murphy, Marie H., Ian Lahart, Angela Carlin, and Elaine Murtagh. "The Effects of Continuous Compared to Accumulated Exercise on Health: A Meta-Analytic Review." Sports Medicine (Auckland, N.Z.) 49, no. 10 (October 2019): 1585–1607.

[←25]

Reitlo, Line Skarsem, Silvana Bucher Sandbakk, Hallgeir Viken, Nils Petter Aspvik, Jan Erik Ingebrigtsen, Xiangchun Tan, Ulrik Wisløff, and Dorthe Stensvold. "Exercise Patterns in Older Adults Instructed to Follow Moderate- or High-Intensity Exercise Protocol - the Generation 100 Study." BMC Geriatrics 18, no. 1 (10 2018): 208.

[←26]

Baechle, Thomas R. Essentials of Strength Training and Conditioning. Champaign, IL: Human Kinetics, 2016.

[←27]

Baechle, Thomas R. Essentials of Strength Training and Conditioning. Champaign, IL: Human Kinetics, 2016.

[←28]

Fransen, Marlene, Sara McConnell, Gabriela Hernandez-Molina, and Stephan Reichenbach. "Exercise for Osteoarthritis of the Hip." The Cochrane Database of Systematic Reviews, no. 4 (April 22, 2014): CD007912. Fransen, Marlene, Sara McConnell, Alison R. Harmer, Martin Van der Esch, Milena Simic, and Kim L. Bennell. "Exercise for Osteoarthritis of the Knee." The Cochrane Database of Systematic Reviews 1 (January 9, 2015): CD004376. Gay, C., A. Chabaud, E. Guilley, and E. Coudeyre. "Educating Patients about the Benefits of Physical Activity and Exercise for Their Hip and Knee Osteoarthritis. Systematic Literature Review." Annals of Physical and Rehabilitation Medicine 59, no. 3 (June 2016): 174–83. Goh, Siew-Li, Monica S. M. Persson, Joanne Stocks, Yunfei Hou, Jianhao Lin, Michelle C. Hall, Michael Doherty, and Weiya Zhang. "Efficacy and Potential Determinants of Exercise Therapy in Knee and Hip Osteoarthritis: A Systematic Review and Meta-Analysis." Annals of Physical and Rehabilitation Medicine 62, no. 5 (September 2019): 356–65. Searle, Angela, Martin Spink, Alan Ho, and Vivienne Chuter. "Exercise Interventions for the Treatment of Chronic Low Back Pain: A Systematic Review and Meta-Analysis of Randomised Controlled Trials." Clinical Rehabilitation 29, no. 12 (December 2015): 1155–67.

[←29]

Liao, Chun-De, Jau-Yih Tsauo, Yen-Tzu Wu, Chin-Pao Cheng, Hui-Chuen Chen, Yi-Ching Huang, Hung-Chou Chen, and Tsan-Hon Liou. "Effects of Protein Supplementation Combined with Resistance Exercise on Body Composition and Physical Function in Older Adults: A Systematic Review and Meta-Analysis." The American Journal of Clinical Nutrition 106, no. 4 (October 2017): 1078–91.

[←30]

Chernoff, Ronni. "Protein and Older Adults." Journal of the American College of Nutrition 23, no. 6 Suppl (December 2004): 627S-630S.

[←31]

Deer, Rachel R., and Elena Volpi. "Protein Intake and Muscle Function in Older Adults." Current Opinion in Clinical Nutrition and Metabolic Care 18, no. 3 (May 2015): 248–53.

[←32]

Whitney, Eleanor Noss, and Sharon Rady Rolfes. Understanding Nutrition, 2019.

[←33]

Newmark, Thomas. "Cases in Visualization for Improved Athletic Performance." Psychiatric Annals 42, no. 10 (October 22, 2012): 385–87.

[←34]

Isaac, Anne R. "Mental Practice — Does It Work in the Field?" The Sport Psychologist 6, no. 2 (June 1, 1992): 192–98.

[←35]

Ranganathan, Vinoth K., Vlodek Siemionow, Jing Z. Liu, Vinod Sahgal, and Guang H. Yue. "From Mental Power to Muscle Power--Gaining Strength by Using the Mind." Neuropsychologia 42, no. 7 (2004): 944–56.

[←36]

Giacobbi, Peter R., Meagan Stabler, Jonathon Stewart, Anna-Marie Jaeschke, Jean L. Siebert, and George A. Kelley. "Guided Imagery for Arthritis and Other Rheumatic Diseases: A Systematic Review of Randomized Controlled Trials." Pain Management Nursing: Official Journal of the American Society of Pain Management Nurses 16, no. 5 (October 2015): 792–803. Malouin, Francine, and Carol L Richards. "Mental Practice for Relearning Locomotor Skills." Physical Therapy 90, no. 2 (February 2010): 240–51.

[←37]

Nicholson, Vaughan P, Justin WL Keogh, and Nancy L Low Choy. "Can a Single Session of Motor Imagery Promote Motor Learning of Locomotion in Older Adults? A Randomized Controlled Trial." Clinical Interventions in Aging 13 (April 23, 2018): 713–22.

[←38]

Grèzes, J., and J. Decety. "Functional Anatomy of Execution, Mental Simulation, Observation, and Verb Generation of Actions: A Meta-Analysis." Human Brain Mapping 12, no. 1 (January 2001): 1–19.

[←39]

Richter, Jeremy, Jenelle N. Gilbert, and Mark Baldis. "Maximizing Strength Training Performance Using Mental Imagery." Strength & Conditioning Journal 34, no. 5 (October 2012): 65–69.

[←40]

Lally P., Van Jaarsveld C.H.M., Potts H.W.W., and Wardle J. 2010. "How are habits formed: Modelling habit formation in the real world". European Journal of Social Psychology. 40 (6): 998-1009.

[←41]

Clear, James. ATOMIC HABITS: An Easy and Proven Way to Build Good Habits and Break Bad Ones. Place of publication not identified: RANDOM House BUSINESS, 2019.

[←42]

Phillips, L. Alison, Pier-Éric Chamberland, Eric B. Hekler, Jessica Abrams, and Miriam H. Eisenberg. 2016. "Intrinsic rewards predict exercise via behavioral intentions for initiators but via habit strength for maintainers". Sport, Exercise, and Performance Psychology. 5 (4): 352-364.

[←43]

Di Domenico, Stefano I., and Richard M. Ryan. "The Emerging Neuroscience of Intrinsic Motivation: A New Frontier in Self-Determination Research." Frontiers in Human Neuroscience 11 (2017): 145.

[←44]

Cuddy, Amy J. C., S. Jack Schultz, and Nathan E. Fosse. "P-Curving a More Comprehensive Body of Research on Postural Feedback Reveals Clear Evidential Value for Power-Posing Effects: Reply to Simmons and Simonsohn (2017)." Psychological Science 29, no. 4 (2018): 656–66.

[←45]

Csikszentmihalyi, Mihaly. Flow: The Psychology of Optimal Experience. New York: Harper [and] Row, 2009.

[←46]

Carretié, L., F. Mercado, M. Tapia, and J. A. Hinojosa. "Emotion, Attention, and the 'Negativity Bias', Studied through Event-Related Potentials." International Journal of Psychophysiology:

Official Journal of the International Organization of Psychophysiology 41, no. 1 (May 2001): 75–85.

[←47]

Vaish, Amrisha, Tobias Grossmann, and Amanda Woodward. "Not All Emotions Are Created Equal: The Negativity Bias in Social-Emotional Development." Psychological Bulletin 134, no. 3 (May 2008): 383–403.

[←48]

Losada, Marcial, and Emily Heaphy. "The Role of Positivity and Connectivity in the Performance of Business Teams: A Nonlinear Dynamics Model." American Behavioral Scientist, July 27, 2016.

[←49]

Gottman, John Mordechai. What Predicts Divorce? The Relationship between Marital Processes and Marital Outcomes, 2009.

[←50]

Cowan, Nelson. "The Magical Mystery Four: How Is Working Memory Capacity Limited, and Why?" Current Directions in Psychological Science 19, no. 1 (February 1, 2010): 51–57.

[←51]

BrainyQuote. "Bonnie Blair Quotes - Citation." Accessed August 29, 2020. https://www.brainyquote.com/citation/quotes/bonnie_blair_204242.